AF270941

No Less Blessed

Seeking God in the Wilderness of
Infertility and Childlessness

Erica F. Mitchell

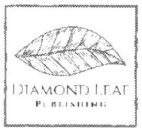

DIAMOND LEAF
PUBLISHING

No Less Blessed: Seeking God in the Wilderness of Infertility and Childlessness

Copyright © 2020 by Erica F. Mitchell

All rights reserved. No part of this publication may be reproduced, stored or transmitted in any form or by any means, electronic, mechanical, photocopying, recording, scanning, or otherwise without prior permission from the author. It is illegal to copy this book, post it to a website, or distribute it by any other means without permission except as provided for by USA copyright law.

Published in Newport News, Virginia, by Diamond Leaf Publishing
First printing 2020

Cover design: Ryan Biore
Author photo: Chun Jea Lee

All Scripture quotations, unless otherwise indicated, are taken from the Holy Bible, New International Version®, NIV®. Copyright ©1973, 1978, 1984, 2011 by Biblica, Inc. Used by permission of Zondervan. All rights reserved worldwide. www.zondervan.comThe "NIV" and "New International Version" are trademarks registered in the United States Patent and Trademark Office by Biblica, Inc.

ESV. Scripture quotations are from the ESV® Bible (The Holy Bible, English Standard Version®), copyright © 2001 by Crossway, a publishing ministry of Good News Publishers. Used by permission. All rights reserved."

GNT. Scripture quotations marked (GNT) are from the Good News Translation in Today's English Version- Second Edition Copyright © 1992 by American Bible Society. Used by Permission.

HCSB. Scripture quotations marked HCSB are taken from the Holman Christian Standard Bible®, Used by Permission HCSB ©1999,2000,2002,2003,2009 Holman Bible Publishers. Holman Christian Standard Bible®, Holman CSB®, and HCSB® are federally registered trademarks of Holman Bible Publishers.

NASB. Scripture taken from the NEW AMERICAN STANDARD BIBLE®, Copyright © 1960,1962,1963,1968,1971,1972,1973,1975,1977,1995 by The Lockman Foundation. Used by permission.

NKJV. Scripture taken from the New King James Version. Copyright © 1982 by Thomas Nelson, Inc. Used by permission. All rights reserved.

NLT. Scripture quotations marked (NLT) are taken from the Holy Bible, New Living Translation, copyright ©1996, 2004, 2015 by Tyndale House Foundation. Used by permission of Tyndale House Publishers, a Division of Tyndale House Ministries, Carol Stream, Illinois 60188. All rights reserved.

All emphases in Scripture quotations have been added by the author.

Print ISBN: 978-0-578-63322-0
ebook ISBN: 978-0-578-63324-4

Library of Congress Control Number: 2020900383

"This is dedicated to the one I love."
I miss you, Papa.

Foreword

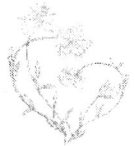

No Less Blessed was one of the most needed books I've read recently. Erica Mitchell's presence, both in person and in word, is most welcome and I am truly privileged to call her a coworker in Christ and friend. For anyone who is looking for someone to genuinely walk with them through the tough questions that come with grief and loss, Erica is the person for you.

Erica Mitchell's No Less Blessed is a very much needed work and offers considerable insight into the deeper questions of faith. With too many writers, pastors, churches peddling pop-spirituality for the masses Mitchell's probe into the depths of our spiritual journey through the lens of loss is sure to uproot feeble brush that has too often left us wanting as we have waded through the more challenging moments and seasons of life.

Her ability to tackle the issue of barrenness by using an unorthodox piece of biblical text (the usual suspects being Hannah, Sarah, Elizabeth, etc.) the wilderness wanderings, is at once refreshing and informative, filling the cracks of pat answers and proof texts that have run dry.

By staying true to the historicity of the wilderness text and not rushing it into today's world, Mitchell expounds biblical truth while uncovering questions and a core that has been shared across all generations; the tension of expedience versus obedience, the definition of blessing and the plague of circumstantial and conditional Christianity.

No Less Blessed was a personally fulfilling book for myself as my wife and I also are treading the same waters of barrenness and loss. Mitchell's unassuming nature and inviting tone allow for the reader who suffers from loss to feel welcomed and to enter those depths, which are often too much to bear alone.

This book is a must-read for any who suffer from loss of any kind and for those who desire to move past superficial clichés and start developing a deeper root of faith.

Yoon Lee
Yoido Full Gospel Church

Contents

Introduction

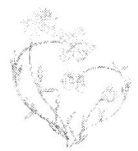

Wife and mother.

The words flow together so seamlessly that you might easily forget a woman can be one and not the other. But I, and millions of women like me, never forget. We're constantly reminded that despite our efforts and prayers, we do not possess a membership to motherhood.

Instead, we learn to circumvent inquiries about whether we have a child. We silently navigate events and environments that celebrate children and parenthood. We plaster an empty smile to hide our heartbreak. We cling to hope as our strength wanes from a prolonged season of infertility and childlessness, and we're discernably weary from the toll it has taken on our emotional, mental, and spiritual health.

For those who have long desired to expand their family but face delays, obstacles, and barriers to parenthood, I stand with you. For over a decade, my husband and I have prayed, cried, and endured hardship alongside you, and we continue to do so to this day. And though I do not wear the crown of motherhood, my journey has not been unfruitful. Infertility has undoubtedly tested my faith in ways that most people do not readily share, but I have also learned that there is strength in my story. Writing this book has helped me to embrace the vulnerability of sharing my experience with the hope that I may be able to provide comfort and insight to others on a similar path.

I believe in the power of testimony and the ability it presents to connect with others in their most obscure places of hurt. It is in our testimony where we identify how we have become "more than conquerors." It is in our testimony where we find God's grace and His distinct love for us.

Since childhood, I have read the Bible and have been inspired and encouraged by the various stories of challenge, hardship, and victory. But my experience with infertility has given me a greater depth of appreciation for how each individual in the Bible managed feelings of frustration, insecurity, doubt, and faith. And each person did not anticipate that their circumstances would qualify or justify them to become leaders and role models; they simply surrendered to God and allowed Him to use their story. As a Christian, I accept their experience as part of my spiritual heritage; and as a woman without a child, they motivate me to share my season of brokenness to encourage the one person who is desperate to read the words on the following pages.

Each chapter begins with a glimpse into my experience with infertility and progresses with the integration of scripture and applicable insight for this adversity. Although I have selected unique moments from my personal journey, I wholeheartedly believe the underlying emotions are universal. You will be able to identify with each experience even if you cannot relate to the specific event. My most sincere hope is that our shared emotional connection resonates such that it allows you to understand the point of view from which I have applied each scripture.

As you read this book, you will see how I endeavored to provide a vital perspective and long-awaited comfort to those struggling in the wilderness of hardship. Each chapter offers a unifying message of how God has not abandoned us and how He hears every prayer and sees every tear, especially when the outcome of our adversity is much different than we expected. Even in our darkest moments, God uses us to share the things that others are desperate to understand and waiting to hear.

Infertility, as with any other hardship, is not something we can endure alone, so I invite you to join me as I present the following chapters. I pray that somewhere within these pages, you find a message that resonates with you and enables you to stand stronger in your own journey or bless others in their hardship. May you fully embrace that you are indeed no less blessed, and may this book be yet another blessing to you.

Chapter 1

Is Anyone There?

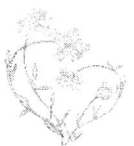

"Because you have seen me, you have believed;
blessed are those who have not seen and yet have believed."

John 20:29

D id you flip to the back of the book?

If I were you, that's what I would have done. I'd want to know more about the author, and I'd be looking for one thing: whether or not she is a mother. I know how that sounds, but it's true. I'd want to see if this book has a similar theme to many of the infertility books on the market—the ones that tell of a difficult, emotional journey that leads to the happy ending for which we are all praying so intently; the journey that ends with a blessing. Well, the spoiler is that I am not one of those authors, and this is not one of those books.

I used to read those books. Each author motivated me, encouraged me, and sustained my hope as I walked through the wilderness of infertility. Their message of endurance resonated with me and fortified my determination to reach the finish line. I celebrated their motherhood victories and renewed my focus to (one day) join them in their winner's circle holding my own child.

But something changed during my season of prolonged waiting. The books started to lose their ability to provide comfort. Where I was once eager to hear the author's testimony, I became indifferent and exhausted by the repetitive message. Eventually, I stopped reading them and donated them to charity. I no longer felt encouraged by their message, and instead, I sat in pain, frustration, and despair, believing nothing would ever provide the consolation and reassurance I desperately needed to hear. Yet because I have always enjoyed reading, it did not take long before I started searching for another book to fill the void.

The more I browsed, the more I saw a pattern. There were two predominant categories of books on infertility: those written by medical professionals, and those written by mothers. Books written by medical professionals shared clinical insight on fertility dysfunctions and provided information on related treatment modalities. And the books written by women reflected upon their infertility testimony of endurance by faith to overcome childlessness with adoption or childbirth. If you toss in a few devotionals and books on alternative remedies, you would have nearly the full catalog of available literature on infertility. There were few resources devoted to the infertility experience in between the medical diagnosis and the miracle testimony. I couldn't find anyone willing to share encouragement from their journey before they received the gift that God had prepared for them, and I was even more disheartened that the prevailing message reinforced the hurtful sentiment that God only loves some women and not others.

I was deeply troubled and wondered why no one was willing to support the prevailing maxim, "God is good all the time, and all the time, God is good," while they were still hurting and waiting. But this was the precise message I needed to hear. I needed reassurance that regardless of whether or not my infertility story ended with the miracle child, God still loved me and was indeed still good. But it seemed as if hardly anyone believed this to be true or had the courage and desire to say this amid their tears and pain. It seemed as if everyone was waiting for confirmation before having the confidence to be an encouragement to someone. But I needed that person, desperately, and I still need that person now.

I need encouragement from the hurting woman who does not have children, but who is still hoping, praying, waiting, and managing her pain.

There are not many books written by men or women testifying to the goodness of God while still in their season of infertility. I wondered whether people were afraid to ask themselves one of the toughest questions regarding their faith—whether they genuinely believed "God is good *all* the time" and whether they could say God was still good *even if* he did not provide them with their prayer request. Then, I came to an awkward and uncomfortable realization— was I afraid to ask myself the same question? Did I believe God was still good in the midst of my pain?

If obedience and willingness to trust God is the measurement of our faith, then what happens when we trust Him only on condition he complies with our requests? What does that say about our faith and what we believe? How do we demonstrate our willingness to trust Him if we do not leave room for His alternative? And what are we saying to men and women when their most fervent prayers are not enough to bring about the picture-perfect ending they have imagined? Some infertile couples wait for years, praying with every ounce of their strength and crying from the depths of their soul, but never experience a miracle pregnancy and childbirth. Yet the available literature on infertility does little to comfort and restore their faith, so they continue to suffer in silence. They struggle with the stigma of not being able to have a child. They wrestle with deep feelings of insecurity and rejection, believing they have not received God's favor. Their relationship with Him begins to fracture, and they start to lose their faith.

Was I willing to trust God and be the author of the book that no one wanted to write?

In a prolonged season of infertility, we need to hear the voice that can speak directly to our struggles and provide empathy for our present sufferings. I am grateful that doctors can speak from a medical perspective. I am grateful that mothers can speak from a place of fulfillment. And I am grateful that other sympathetic authors have written from indirect experience. But there is a desperate need for this void to be filled by authors who can proclaim that God is just as good in the middle of the story as He is at the end of the chapter. When we truly believe that God is good, we believe that He is good even if the ending looks radically different than how we have imagined and prayed. When we truly believe that God is good, we believe that there is power in our testimony to both encourage someone and identify an opportunity to reach the needs of an overlooked community.

When we truly believe that God is good, we trust Him to sustain us as we write our first book with tears in our eyes.

I am the author that no one wanted to be. I am in the middle of my season of infertility, and I still hope, wait, and pray for God to provide closure to my story. But I have learned quite a few things that I pray will be an encouragement to those who, like me, have started flipping to the back of the book. I want you to know that you are "no less blessed" than those who have received your heart's desire. I want you to know when you surrender to God, you are not giving up hope. I want you to know when you don't see the value of your testimony in the middle of your storm, you will stumble in your faith. I want you to know you are the author for whom you have been waiting. And I want you to believe that God is good, both in the big picture blessing and in the moment-by-moment grace, because it is the moment-by-moment grace that leads you to the place God has prepared for you.

But mostly, I want you to know that the book you are searching for is probably already in your possession. I believe that book to be the Bible. It provides comfort and reassurance and just takes prayer, perspective, and reflection to be able to receive the healing and insight found within its pages. When we look to the Bible, we witness hundreds of stories from people whose lives were riddled with challenge and hardship, but who overcame their hurt and pain because of the God who was present with them. That is the foundation of the encouragement that we must embrace during our season of waiting.

Insight from the Scriptures

This book does not represent the first time I've sought biblical insight for my experience with infertility. To be fair, there are plenty of Christian infertility books already on the market. But the common theme behind the available resources is that many rely on the literal infertility stories of the Bible. The most prominently referenced stories are those of Sarah, Hannah, Rachel, and Elizabeth. Let's do a quick review of their narratives.

Sarah *(Genesis 15-21)*

God made a promise to Sarah's husband, Abraham, that He would make Abraham "into a great nation." At the time, Abraham and Sarah did not have children. After several years of infertility, Sarah became impatient and devised a plan for Abraham to sleep with her servant, Hagar, who birthed him a son. Yet, despite Sarah's intervention, God remained faithful to his word, and Sarah ultimately conceived her son, Isaac.

Hannah *(1 Samuel 1)*

Hannah was one of two wives to Elkanah. His second wife, Peninnah, was described as Hannah's rival because she was able to birth multiple children while Hannah had none. Hannah was in deep anguish and wept and prayed fervently to the Lord, asking him for a child. In exchange, she vowed to dedicate the child to the Lord's service. A priest noticed Hannah and blessed her, and God granted Hannah's request. Hannah became pregnant and she remained faithful to her vow by dedicating her son, Samuel, to a life of serving the Lord.

Rachel *(Genesis 29-30)*

Rachel and her sister, Leah, were both married to Jacob. Although Jacob loved and favored Rachel over Leah, Rachel was unable to conceive a child while her sister was able to have multiple children. Rachel became jealous (and competitive) and used her servant to conceive children with Jacob. Leah and her servant conceived additional children, then Rachel finally conceived a child—her son Joseph.

Elizabeth *(Luke 1)*

Elizabeth and her husband, Zechariah, were righteous in the sight of God, and faithfully observed his word. They did not have children and were not of childbearing age. Zechariah was approached by an angel of the Lord who declared that his wife would become pregnant with a son who would be filled with the Holy Spirit. Elizabeth became pregnant and gave birth to her son, John.

Additional narratives of infertility can be found in the Bible if you also include the stories of Abimelech's wife and servants, Rebekah, Manoah's wife, the Shunammite woman, and Michal.

Abimelek's household *(Genesis 20)*

Abimelek was the King of Gerar. He integrated Sarah (mentioned above) into his harem when he was deceived into believing she was Abraham's sister instead of his wife. When God told Abimelek that Sarah was indeed a married woman, Abimelek released her. Abraham prayed to God, and God restored fertility to Abimelek and his household.

Rebekah *(Genesis 25:19-26)*

Isaac, the son of Abraham and Sarah, married Rebekah and prayed to the Lord because Rebekah was childless. Rebekah conceived and birthed twin boys, Jacob and Esau.

Manoah's wife *(Judges 25)*

Manoah's wife was childless until an angel of the Lord appeared to her and informed her that she would become pregnant. She was instructed to abstain from wine, fermented drink, unclean food, and never cut the child's hair. She became pregnant and gave birth to a son whom she named Samson.

The Shunammite woman *(2 Kings 4:8-41)*

An affluent woman from Shunem was hospitable to the prophet Elisha, who, in turn, prophesied that she would have a son.

Despite her husband's old age and her own hesitation to believe the prophecy, she gave birth to a son in the following year.

Michal *(2 Samuel 6)*

Michal was the daughter of King Saul and the first wife of David. When David became king and brought the ark of the covenant to Jerusalem, he danced with all of his might before the Lord. Michal watched him from a window with contempt, believing that he was being vulgar and inappropriate because his behavior seemed outlandish and his appearance half-naked. David rebuked her for criticizing his praise dancing for the Lord, and she never had children.

Each narrative appropriately reflects the identity of God as the giver of life. Since each woman (except Michal) ultimately became pregnant, many people conclude that the longer you wait and the harder you pray that you, too, will become pregnant.

While I wholeheartedly support that nothing is impossible with God and that He can indeed miraculously make the barren woman a mother, I also know that He loves each of us immensely. The simple conclusion to "pray harder, wait longer, and then you will become pregnant" can be especially hurtful to women who pray and cry with all of their strength, yet never birth a child. It sends the message that their prayers were not good enough, or that there was some spiritual deficit they personally failed to overcome in persuading God to open their womb. Neither of these insinuations is an accurate representation of God's love for them. I personally know many women who arrived at the end of their window of fertility (or whose medical circumstances precluded them from birthing a child), and I witnessed how this message severely wounded their faith and relationship with God. This message, in its simplicity, does not reinforce the love that God has for each man and woman irrespective of their ability to become mothers and fathers. This message, albeit unintentionally, redirects the goodness of God to the gift of childbirth instead of the gift of spiritual intimacy and salvation.

The "pray harder, wait longer" mantra feels very dismissive of the ongoing spiritual struggle that men and women must endure. The intense emotions that accompany a prolonged season of infertility can make for a very challenging experience. Men and women must manage recurring disappointment, repeated frustration, indescribable loss, profound yearning, and a desert of uncertainty. It is here, with these challenges, where the Bible is most helpful in comforting and guiding infertile couples.

Instead of limiting encouragement to the literal biblical narratives of fertility, I have found incredible insight from a different Bible story. There are clear similarities in the emotional experience and thought processes between the struggle of navigating through infertility and the hardships encountered by the Israelites as they traversed the wilderness. This book will examine significant lessons from the journey of the Israelites as recorded in Exodus 13 – Deuteronomy 34. I'll demonstrate how each lesson has provided discernment and value to my own journey. Each of the following chapters opens with a glimpse into a very personal, but typical, experience with infertility, and I'll connect this experience to a lesson from the Israelite narrative. Their story adds comforting depth and sound insight to the guidance of merely praying and waiting, and is a fresh approach to infertility beyond the frequently referenced biblical accounts. I sincerely hope that each chapter helps you broaden your view, restore your faith, and renew your conviction to believe you are "no less blessed" than the men and women who have received your heart's desire.

In Summary

- ❀ The majority of infertility books approach the topic from a medical perspective or are written by mothers who have overcome infertility by miracle pregnancy and adoption. There are few books written that speak to the goodness of God amid infertility and without having first received the blessing of a child.

- ❀ Many Christian books on infertility rely on the fertility narratives of the Bible. Most of the infertility narratives in the Bible conclude with a miracle pregnancy; thus, Christian literature often concludes that couples must simply pray harder and wait longer to conquer infertility and receive a miracle pregnancy. This message can be especially heartbreaking and spiritually defeating for couples that never conceive or sustain a pregnancy.

- ❀ By examining the biblical narrative of the Israelites journey through the wilderness, infertile couples will notice the emotional and mental similarities to navigating through infertility. This particular narrative adds additional depth and perspective to the "pray harder and wait longer" advice frequently given to infertile couples, and is quintessential to restoring and maintaining their faith and relationship with God.

Chapter 2

Rerouting

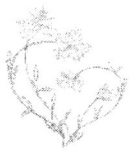

When you walk, your steps will not be hampered;
when you run, you will not stumble.

Proverbs 4:12

Five...Four...Three...Two...One...

And here we go.

It never fails. Anytime I'm with a group of my peers, I have a silent countdown of how long it takes before the conversation changes to the latest challenge they're facing with their children. It doesn't bother me; it just happens so frequently I've nearly grown numb to it. But the longer they talk, the less I have to contribute. I tend to withdraw and remain quiet, silently nodding and smiling. I've gotten into the habit of daydreaming or mentally disengaging so I do not become too emotionally vulnerable. I try to look at my phone or excuse myself altogether if it becomes an extended conversation about raising children. I don't want them to feel uncomfortable, but at the same time, I don't want to torture myself either. I don't want to make the mistake of saying something that elicits the soul-crushing response of "You're not a mother, you wouldn't understand".

It's not hard for me to remember that 1 in 8 couples experience infertility[1]. That means there's a pretty strong chance I'll be in a group conversation that discusses parenthood while being the only one who doesn't have kids. As the 1 in 8, I know quite well how infertility creates an atmosphere of exclusion and the unique position of being the exception without feeling exceptional. It can distort your identity and affect your self-esteem.

It's like winning the rejection lottery.

I received a diagnosis for the underlying condition of my infertility more than 15 years ago. I remember how the nurse practitioner thoughtlessly glanced at my medical chart, visually assessed my physical features, and then bluntly informed me that I had a common hormonal disorder. She shrugged aside any concerns I had about this new diagnosis and said it would only be an issue when I wanted to get pregnant. But, because I was young and unmarried, she did not desire to discuss the condition in detail.

For years, I researched my condition and joined online forums that promoted awareness and education. I continued to ask medical professionals about it, but they continued to silence me because they considered me to be too young to have a legitimate concern. Even after I got married and struggled to conceive, doctors constantly ignored and belittled my inquiries about how I could overcome my medical challenges. To them, I was always too young to be worried,

---

[1] RESOLVE: The National Infertility Association, "Fast Facts," resolve.org, February 2020, https://resolve.org/infertility-101/what-is-infertility/fast-facts.

too much of a newlywed to want to expand my family, and too much of an "internet physician" to substantiate that I had valid concerns.

So, nearly 11 years into my marriage, I've still never experienced the joy of a positive pregnancy test or even the tragic loss of miscarriage. My womb has simply remained eerily silent. I've seen multiple fertility specialists and listened to their confident, albeit costly, promises of success. I've taken pills and injections to trigger biological processes that should have occurred naturally. I've learned the crazy acronym language of infertility, such as TTC, BFN, ART, and DH (i.e., trying to conceive, big fat negative [pregnancy test], assisted reproductive technology, and my "dear husband"). I've ridden the roller coaster of foster care and adoption and had more disappointments than I care to remember.

It's just been a long road.

And one of the hardest things about infertility is reconciling that life is not going "according to plan." There's a not-so-silent expectation that once you get married, you're supposed to have children. In fact, the process of going from childfree to parent presents itself as so straightforward and uncomplicated that it warrants prevention against unanticipated pregnancy more so than overcoming fertility challenges.

Even though I knew I would have trouble getting pregnant, I never imagined the journey would be this long or this hard. The experience has felt quite sad, lonely, and even embarrassing at times. It's the journey through infertility that has impacted me even more than the identity of being a non-parent. The experience is fully wrought with hope and heartbreak, tears and trauma, disappointment and frustration, loss and longing, waiting, praying, and wandering. It's why I've found comfort in the biblical narrative of the Israelites as they roamed the wilderness to their promised land. Their long journey feels comparable to my prolonged season of infertility and childlessness. Their experience parallels the fear, frustration, and uncertainty that couples endure in a season of adversity and hardship.

Insight from the Scriptures

The journey of the Israelites begins in Exodus 12:31 when Pharaoh summons Moses and Aaron to declare that the Israelites and their families are free to leave Egypt. The Israelites had been living in Egypt for 430 years, where they endured slavery and captivity. Notice the first parallel between their story and our infertility narrative as they embark upon their journey to the land that God promised to them. Exodus 13:17-18 states,

*"When Pharaoh let the people go, God did not lead them on the road through the Philistine country, **though that was shorter**. For God said, 'If they face war, they might change their minds and return to Egypt.' So God led the people around by the desert road toward the Red Sea. The Israelites went up out of Egypt ready for battle."*

The Israelites were not led by the shortest, most direct, and obvious path to their destination. Likewise, infertility impedes our direct path to parenthood. Infertility complicates a process that should occur naturally and without much effort. It causes us to wait longer, take an alternate route, or reconsider our final destination altogether.

Although infertility may feel like punishment, we have to trust that God is not punishing us with a lengthy journey, just as he did not lead the Israelites out of Egypt using a longer route based on a whim. To the Israelites, he may have seemed like he was indifferent to the 430 years they endured in bondage by not leading them to the promised land as quickly as possible. But what they could not see was that He was being merciful, preparing their minds and helping them to avoid war with the Philistines. Had the Israelites encountered conflict, God knew they would have been discouraged and returned to Egypt.

While I would never be so foolish and cruel to say that God causes infertility, miscarriage, or pregnancy loss, this early lesson from the Israelites makes evident that He sees obstacles on our path before we even encounter them. And He demonstrates that sometimes an obstacle is so tough that, in His wisdom, he redirects us away from it without us even knowing about it.

Nonetheless, there is still a hurtful assumption by many that God explicitly causes us to endure infertility because it is either not in His will for us to ever become parents, or it is a punishment for some spiritual deficit that we have not reconciled. When fertility prayers seemingly go unanswered, men and women silently chastise and criticize themselves for being unworthy or not good enough to receive God's gift of conception and childbirth. This self-flagellation is not necessary. Romans 3:23-24 tells us that we all have fallen short of God's glory. If every sin led to infertility, then no one would have children. The fact that some people struggle to have children while others have no such challenge does not indicate that God has a personal vendetta against specific people. Instead, it is a reflection of the fallen, broken world in which we live. No one escapes life unscathed by deep hurt, pain, and desire. Our prayers for children go to the same God that hears prayers for food, housing, healing, and countless other requests. It is not His will that any of us should suffer in vain, just as it was not His will for the Israelites to be discouraged by a conflict with the Philistines on the direct path out of Egypt.

The Bible says that there were 600,000 Israelite men on the journey, excluding women, children, and other people (Exodus 12:37-

38). There must have been at least a few people in the multitude that did not understand the reason behind the direction they were traveling. Similarly, I don't pretend to know why 1 in 8 couples experience infertility, but I do know there was a purpose to the route of the Israelites:

God used this alternate route as a major part of their story.

The alternative path towards the Red Sea positioned the Israelites to witness one of the greatest miracles described in the Bible.

Exodus 14:5-29 describes the event of the Israelites being fully delivered from Pharaoh and his army. When the Israelites left Egypt and Pharaoh realized the impact of losing their free (slave) labor, he changed his mind about their freedom and decided to pursue them with his army. The Israelites saw the Egyptian army and began to panic and worry, but Moses reassured them by saying,

"Do not be afraid. Stand firm and you will see the deliverance the Lord will bring you today. The Egyptians you see today you will never see again. The Lord will fight for you; you need only to be still" (Exodus 14:13-14).

As the angel of the Lord stood in between the Egyptian army and Israel, Moses stretched his hand over the sea, and the Lord divided the sea with a strong wind. The Israelites were able to walk on dry land in between two walls of water. When Pharoah's army pursued them, the Lord commanded Moses to stretch his hand back over the sea. The waters flowed back into place, drowning the entire army. But the Israelites made it safely to the other side of the sea.

They had witnessed a great miracle and a manifestation of the power and protection of the Lord. However, a few days after celebrating this great victory and singing a song of praise to the Lord, the Israelites grew bitter about their circumstances, and this eventually become a defining characteristic of their entire journey. They failed to remember the incredible illustration of God's power and demonstration of His love, concern, and protection over them; and they continued to disregard the blessings they received throughout the journey.

During our lifetime, we will undoubtedly encounter an incredible miracle—something that indicates to us that God is with us; something that transcends circumstance and serendipity; something that is unique to our situation. It may not be as literal as dividing the sea, but it will be something that has a significant impact on our life. Whatever it may be, my challenge to you is to remember it. Do not stand in awe and only praise God in the moment, but continuously reflect upon it and give thanks. Hold on to that memory, preserving its influence over your life and faith, and allowing it to serve as encouragement in sustaining you through the difficult roads of your journey.

We may wonder to ourselves how the Israelites could ever harbor any bitterness or doubt towards God after personally witnessing such a significant event, but the reality is that we do it all the time. Our praise and enthusiasm fade when hardship appears. Infertility has the uncanny ability to hoard our thoughts and direct our attention to what we do not have, and it becomes harder and harder to remember and appreciate the majestic things we have witnessed in our own life.

We cannot allow our pain, fear, and prayers for fertility to silence our heart of gratitude and immobilize us from going where God is guiding us to go.

One of the most interesting similarities between the narrative of the Israelites at the Red Sea and our own experience with infertility is found in Exodus 14:15. The Lord says to Moses, "Why are you crying out to me? Tell the Israelites to move on." The Lord makes this statement immediately after Moses encourages the Israelites to be still and see the deliverance of the Lord. His encouragement is very similar to the common advice that many well-intentioned friends and family members provide to us in our season of infertility—"pray harder and keep waiting." Yes, we should absolutely 'pray without ceasing,' 'pray incessantly,' 'be faithful in prayer,' and continue to follow the instruction of the many scriptures that coach us in sustaining our prayer relationship with God, but we also have a momentum we must maintain in following God as we journey along this alternate path. God was not scolding Moses to stop praying, or even that He required more prayer to fuel His mighty miracle; instead, it was a directive to keep moving!

Prayer is vital to our faith, but we cannot use it as an excuse to stop once God has given us our 'marching orders.' Even Hannah, who was overcome with infertility grief, prayed in anguish until Eli the priest advised her to "go in peace," at which time she went on her way, ate, and no longer appeared distressed (1 Samuel 1:12-18). Hannah did not linger, nor did she continue to mope about her situation. She was given her 'marching orders,' and she kept moving.

I speak from experience in acknowledging that this is hard. It's hard to keep moving when you don't know specifically what God is doing with your situation. It's hard to keep moving with what God has given you when you still have questions or when you feel emotionally paralyzed. But how ironic is it that the image that comes to my mind is a weeping child who has been given direction that he does not emotionally understand. I imagine that he either lays on the floor wailing and having a tantrum, or that he complies with the request, albeit with tears and sniffling. I would like to believe that, in a spiritual sense, I am the child that is sniffling and complying with what God has told me to do. But I'd be untruthful if I didn't acknowledge that I have had more than a few spiritual temper-tantrums. However, I am so grateful that the Lord is a "compassionate and gracious God, slow to anger, abounding in love and faithfulness" (Psalm 86:15). Even my temper-tantrums have not disqualified me from receiving the good things He has in store for me.

Infertility, like every other challenge, requires us to walk in faith, and faith is a muscle that we must continue to flex for the entirety of our lives. When our path takes an alternate route, we may flex our faith with a smile, but many times we will flex our faith with tears. And even during the times we flex our faith after a tantrum, our bucket of humility and remorse can reach into God's deep well of mercy and forgiveness. We must continue to refresh and remind ourselves that His relationship with us is built from love, not punishment. We must believe that He is compassionate and faithful to us, even when we are rerouted.

In Summary

※ Infertility leads us down an alternate path. Just as the Israelites were not guided down a direct path, infertility causes us to travel an indirect path to parenthood. But God demonstrated through the Israelites that He does not send us down an alternate path without purpose and without His presence.

※ An important responsibility in our infertility journey is to recall and reflect on the major things that God is doing in our life. The Israelites disregarded the miracle at the Red Sea as soon as they were faced with adversity. We cannot allow the blessings and miracles that are occurring in our life to be overshadowed by the hardship of infertility. We must honor them, keep them in remembrance, and continuously give praise for them because they will become a crucial component of our journey.

❋ We cannot allow our pain or fear to keep us from moving and maintaining momentum with God. Prayer is vital to our faith and our communication with God, but we cannot use it as an excuse to stop moving when we have been given direction from the Lord.

Chapter 3

Fruitful

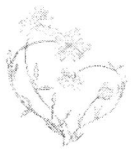

*I would have despaired unless I had believed that
I would see the goodness of the Lord in the land of the living.*

Psalm 27:13 (NASB)

I 'm dangerous on the internet.

I'm the type of person where one thought leads to another, one curious question births an endless stream of inquiries. At any given moment, you'll find me researching something on my phone, tablet, or computer; it doesn't matter. I can get lost for hours perusing Google, reading articles, saving websites, and daydreaming about any and everything.

So it's no surprise that as I was writing a book on infertility, I found myself back on adoption websites. What started as innocent research evolved into an emotional investment in the multiple contact submission forms I completed to request additional information about their services. I wanted to know whether each agency would allow me to use their services. But 24-hours later, I woke up to an inbox full of rejection letters. Because of the unique circumstances of where we lived, no one was willing to work with us. We were a military family stationed abroad, and despite our status as U.S. citizens with a Virginia residency, each agency encouraged me to try again in a few years once we returned to the States.

I wish I could say that I was able to put life on pause while I worked on this book—that I was not constantly tending to my own hopes for parenthood recovering from sadness while writing a book to encourage others. But that would be far from accurate. As I write, my closest friends are celebrating their pregnancy, birth, and adoption announcements; I inched another year closer to the end of my window of fertility, and I am struggling to get through one of the hardest Mother's Day weekends I have ever had to endure.

This project has not been easy by any means. Some days I am the author, armed with inspiration and insight, and some days I am the audience, desperate to hear something to help me through a tough moment and receive a fresh perspective. I am eager to get to the end of this book, both for my own sense of completion and for the support I know it will provide. But it's a slow process that seems to creeps along just one day at a time.

I find the strength to keep going because I know that God knows all of the spiritual, intellectual, physical, and emotional resources that I need to bring this book to completion. I keep trekking along because I envision how it would feel to be finished and how many people this book could comfort. It doesn't make my current challenges hurt any less; it just gives me something to do, something to focus on, and an amazing hope to look forward to so that I don't become overwhelmed and disheartened.

In his faithfulness, God did the same for the Israelites.

Three months after the Israelites left Egypt, they encamped in the desert in front of Mount Sinai. Let's examine a few scenes from Exodus 19-31, where God is speaking to Moses. I want to show you God's compassion, and how He provided it to the Israelites during their journey, just as He continues to demonstrate compassion for our own experience.

Insight from the Scriptures

God promised to bring the Israelites to a land flowing with milk and honey, but several enemies were occupying the promised land. God told Moses that He would drive the enemies out of the way and that the enemies would "turn their backs and run" (Ex. 23:27). However, in Exodus 23:29-30 God says,

> *"But I will not drive them out in a single year,*
> *because the land would become desolate and the*
> *wild animals too numerous for you. Little by little*
> *I will drive them out before you, until you have*
> *increased enough to take possession of the land."*

God was not concerned that the Israelites would struggle in their conflict with the enemy (He would handle that Himself); He was concerned that the territory was too vast for the Israelites to manage effectively. God was saying their success would come incrementally. He knew the size of the land would not be helpful for the fledgling nation of Israel. Instead, He would drive out the enemies "little by little" to allow the Israelites the opportunity to grow, strengthen themselves, and prepare to accept added responsibility.

Many of us are familiar with the popular saying, "God will not put more on you than you can bear." If you look for this statement quoted verbatim in the Bible, you will not find it. The closest resemblance is found in 1 Corinthians 10:13 where Paul writes,

"No temptation has overtaken you except what
is common to mankind. And God is faithful;
he will not let you be tempted beyond what
you can bear. But when you are tempted, he will
also provide a way out so that you can endure it."

Paul was writing specifically about the temptation to sin and not about general hardship, yet it still demonstrates God's benevolence and foresight. Even though we do not have a direct scripture that states God will not overwhelm us, this is the precise compassion that He had for the Israelites during their journey. First, He led them down an alternate path so that they would not encounter war with the Philistines and retreat back into bondage in Egypt (Exodus 13:17). Now, we see that God would not instantaneously eradicate the enemies from the promised land because He did not want the Israelites to become overwhelmed by the vastness of the land that awaited them.

Am I saying that God allows our season of infertility because he thinks we are incapable of parenthood? Absolutely not! I don't believe that at all, especially since there are plenty of men and women who have become parents despite their level of maturity or readiness. But what I do believe is that God is all-knowing. He knew what the Israelites would encounter. He knew how the Israelites would struggle. And most importantly, He knew what He needed to do for them. They didn't know the big picture or the best way through the circumstances that awaited them, but God knew. It's the same for us.

In His compassion, God hears every one of our prayers, sees our tears, and feels our pain. He knows what to do while we are still hoping, waiting, and praying.

That's why I appreciate the narrative of the Israelites. I feel like I can relate to how the Israelites must have felt on their journey. I'm sure there were more than a few men and women who were tired, frustrated, and clueless about what was happening, which is precisely how infertility makes me feel at times. There is so much insight we can gain from examining their story. We can learn from their actions, both what they did and what they should have done. And we can learn from what God was doing amid their uncertainty.

God knew the best path to guide the Israelites to the promised land. He knew what challenges they would face and what resources they would need. He also knew this was their opportunity to strengthen and solidify themselves as His chosen nation. He gave Moses detailed laws and commandments and made a covenant with the Israelites. He also provided precise instructions on the building of the tabernacle and its elements. In Exodus 31:2-6 the Lord says to Moses,

"See, I have chosen Bezalel son of Uri, the son of Hur,
of the tribe of Judah, and I have filled him with the
Spirit of God, with wisdom, with understanding, with
knowledge and with all kinds of skills-- to make artistic
designs for work in gold, silver, and bronze, to cut and
set stones, to work in wood, and to engage in all kinds
of crafts. Moreover, I have appointed Oholiab son of
Ahisamak, of the tribe of Dan, to help him. Also,
I have given ability to all the skilled workers to
make everything I have commanded you..."

Their season of waiting was not intended to be a season of idleness. God gave them an assignment and also bestowed upon them the gifts, talents, and abilities to bring His tabernacle to fruition. He wanted the Israelites not just to trust and follow Him but to stay active in His service as well.

I can personally attest that staying active during a waiting period is one of the best ways to pass the time. My husband has faithfully served as an active duty sailor in the United States Navy for over 19 years. As a military wife, I have had to say goodbye to him on more occasions than I can count. When he leaves for deployment and other mission-essential assignments, I have learned that the best way to pass the time is to focus on projects and social companionship to keep myself busy and comforted while he is away. This is considerably different from my days as a newlywed when I sulked around the house, watching the clock, and frequently checking my email and social media accounts waiting to hear from him. That only made the waiting much longer and more difficult. In fact, military personnel (including my husband) will tell you when their spouse is miserable, it's more challenging for them to focus on their job, safety, and mission. They want to know they are missed and you are thinking of them and praying for them, but they also want to know that you, yourself, are staying active and doing well. When my husband is away and he calls home, our best conversations are the ones where we can share good news. We don't compete about 'who has it worse;' instead, we talk about what we have been able to do despite our distance and the creative ways we were able to resolve some individual challenge. We still miss each other tremendously, but we have learned that this cannot be the focus of each and every phone call for the duration of his absence.

As Christians, this mindset to stay active is not only good for our emotional health, but it is fundamental to our spiritual health as well.

Jesus gave us the most important assignment in Matthew 28:19-20 where he says,

> *"Therefore go and make disciples of all nations,*
> *baptizing them in the name of the Father and of*
> *the Son and of the Holy Spirit, and teaching them to*
> *obey everything I have commanded you. And surely*
> *I am with you always, to the very end of the age."*

We have been given the commission to preach and teach the things we have learned from Jesus. What does this specifically have to do with infertility? Nothing, and everything. Preaching the gospel does not necessarily improve our fertility outcomes, but we can absolutely be spiritually fruitful *because* of our infertility.

One of the most compelling motivations fueling my desire to complete this book is seeing the increasing number of men and women who have hardened their hearts and are distancing themselves from God—either because their season of infertility concluded without a child or their delay has been so long that they're unsure whether He is listening or if He even exists at all. It truly breaks my heart to know that there are so few resources for people who are desperate to hear scriptural encouragement through the lens of infertility that differs from the dismissive statements of "just wait," "just pray," or "just adopt." There is a desperate need to hear encouragement from people who can empathize with infertility, miscarriage, pregnancy loss, and adoption disruption. There is a need to build the kingdom with stories such as yours. There is a desperate need to hear about the goodness of God and reassurance of his promises from people like you, especially while still in your season of infertility.

The Lord told Moses that he filled Bezalel with "the Spirit of God, with wisdom, with understanding, with knowledge and with all kinds of skills" to enable him to complete the crafting required to build the tabernacle and its elements (Ex. 31:3). We, too, are qualified. We have been empowered to do the things that Jesus has commissioned us to do. Jesus has provided us with the Holy Spirit. Jesus says,

> *"If you love me, keep my commands. And I will ask the Father, and he will give you another advocate to help you and be with you forever-- the Spirit of truth. The world cannot accept him, because it neither sees him nor knows him. But you know him, for he lives with you and will be in you... But the Advocate, the Holy Spirit, whom the Father will send in my name, will teach you all things and will remind you of everything I have said to you."*
> *(John 14:15-17, 26)*

As believers and followers of Jesus Christ, we have been given the Holy Spirit. Just as Bezalel received what he needed for his construction assignment, we, too, received what we need to build the kingdom. The Holy Spirit will empower us with the wisdom, understanding, and the skills to perform whatever work we have been invited to do. In 1 Corinthians 12:4-11 (ESV), Paul writes,

> *"Now there are varieties of gifts, but the same Spirit; and there are varieties of service, but the same Lord; and there are varieties of activities, but it is the same God who empowers them all in everyone. To each is given the manifestation of the Spirit for the common*

good. For to one is given through the Spirit the utterance of wisdom, and to another the utterance of knowledge according to the same Spirit, to another faith by the same Spirit, to another gifts of healing by the one Spirit, to another the working of miracles, to another prophecy, to another the ability to distinguish between spirits, to another various kinds of tongues, to another the interpretation of tongues. All these are empowered by one and the same Spirit, who apportions to each one individually as he wills."

Yes, we have been given spiritual gifts along with our unique God-given talents. We are indeed God's workmanship, created to do the good work that he has prepared for us (Ephesians 2:10 NASB). Whether that good work is for you to build the kingdom through wisdom and empathy from your experience with infertility, or to focus on a different area, we must build nonetheless.

We cannot lose sight of the truth that our individual experiences occur within the context of a larger story. God did not merely desire to lead the Israelites from slavery to a land of freedom; their storyline occurs within the context of a larger narrative to deliver humanity from the bondage of sin to a kingdom free from sin, death, and destruction. Our infertility experience is the same.

There is so much more to what God is trying to do for us beyond our desire to build a family. We are still living within the context of what Jesus is doing to shepherd us to our true 'promised land.' Even the biblical narratives of infertility occur within the context of God's plan for salvation and redemption. Whether it was to usher in an ancestor within the genealogy of Christ, or to birth a child with a meaningful impact on the framework of scripture, nothing occurred outside of the blueprint of God's plan for humankind.

That's really heavy, I know.

And I know that some people will not find that to be comforting for their pain at all. But I hope you can see how *empowering* it can be.

Infertility does not have to be the isolating blemish of our lives; rather, it can be the tool we use to connect with other brokenhearted people to preach and teach the goodness of God. Imagine the faith you can restore or build by helping people see God's love by empathizing with the unique pain that many of us silently endure. Or, imagine how well you can persist in your season of waiting by being faithful to the commission that Jesus has given us. In either scenario, heaven is waiting to rejoice for the one person that you can lead back to the arms of God (Luke 15:7). Let's not be so overwhelmed that we stop doing the work that God has given us to do. In doing this, infertility cannot and will not win.

In Summary

- God knows what we need during this difficult time. He knows where we struggle, and he knows the best way to shepherd us to our destination. He demonstrates his compassion even when we don't know it.

- Just as God gave the Israelites work to do during their journey, we, too, have been commissioned to build the kingdom during our journey through infertility. One of the best ways to persevere through a season of waiting is to remain active.

- We have been given the Holy Spirit to empower us with wisdom, understanding, knowledge, and skills to do the work that God has prepared for us to do. Infertility (and miscarriage, pregnancy loss, adoption disruption, etc.) can be the opportunity that we use to connect with others who are hurting and struggling in their faith. Or, we can use the power of the Holy Spirit to stay active in whatever kingdom-building work we have been called to do. Despite our infertility, we must remain fruitful.

Chapter 4

Drift

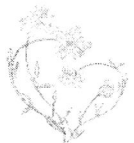

For he has not despised or scorned
the suffering of the afflicted one;
he has not hidden his face from him
but has listened to his cry for help.

Psalms 22:24

I couldn't deny that God had given her the gift of motherhood.

I had decided to meet a friend one evening for a walk, and during our casual conversation, the topic veered to our shared experience with infertility. She had wrestled with infertility for a few years before miraculously becoming pregnant with not one, but two babies. Her advice to me? "Tell God to make you a mother."

We continued walking with a noticeable silence between us. She was allowing her words to sink in, and I was quietly contemplating whether her comment was outrageous or if I, indeed, was not praying with enough confidence. She had shared the story of how she used her conviction to tell God what He was going to do for her, and as a result, she was now the proud mother of two beautiful children. She concluded that my barrenness was a result of my weakness, and if I really wanted to be a mother, then I needed to be bold and demand that God make it happen.

I felt defeated and didn't have a response for her.

Of all the debatable things that have been advised to me during my season of infertility, that one hurt the most because it came from someone who could relate to my pain. Although she could remember her infertility experience, she had lost her sensitivity to how hurtful certain statements can be. And I'm not sure if our friendship ever has - or ever will, recover.

My husband and I had waited, prayed passionately, and tried to become parents by multiple different avenues. Ten years of cycling between anticipation and disappointment is a long time by anyone's measurement. Had I started to feel like a failure? Absolutely. I couldn't figure out what I was doing (or not doing) in my spiritual relationship that resulted in this prolonged season of infertility. It seemed like somehow everyone else had it all figured out; everyone else had become a parent in a fraction of the time it was taking me to reach this milestone. I wondered if she was right. It's not like it was the first time I had heard a comment like that. "You're not praying hard enough" is one of the most commonly unsolicited statements a woman will hear during a season of infertility. Was God ignoring me? Was he abandoning me because he saw me as pathetic?

For years I suppressed these questions and didn't think about them again until I attended a weekend women's retreat. The theme of the retreat focused on becoming your authentic self by releasing unnecessary baggage. I sat through each workshop, impressed with the presenters, but unmoved by the content until we reached a session on the topic of forgiveness. The presenter instructed the audience to muster the courage to face our deepest pain by writing a symbolic letter to the person who hurt us. The goal was to get us to move past unhealed wounds.

After receiving her instructions, the room fell silent except for the soft music gently playing in the background. As the participants began to write their letters, their tears started to fall and you could hear sniffling. As the sniffling increased to sobbing, I stared at my blank sheet of paper, wondering what I should do. I didn't have anyone to forgive. I already felt unburdened ... until I got real with myself.

Erica, nothing is hurting you? Really?

Those suppressed thoughts about feeling ignored and abandoned by God came flooding back. I didn't realize how hurt I had become from believing God saw me as weak and pathetic. I didn't believe He truly cared about me. I would readily tell anyone that I was a Christian, but I didn't realize how far I had drifted in the sincerity of my faith. I was so angry about this prolonged season of waiting and didn't understand why God was punishing me.

I was in anguish as I came face-to-face with the bitterness that I had silently harbored for all of the years of unanswered prayers, all the negative pregnancy test results, all the celebrations and congratulations that I had endured for other women while wondering when it would be my turn, and the unsuccessful attempts at adoption that I so confidently believed God would bless. My honest truth was that I was mad at God.

Prolonged waiting can lead to frustration, and frustration can tempt you to drift away from God. Do we see this happen with the Israelites?

Definitely.

Insight from the Scriptures

As if witnessing the parting of the Red Sea wasn't enough, the Israelites received yet another opportunity to observe God's power and dominion.

In Exodus 19:16-19, Moses leads the people to the foot of Mount Sinai to meet with God. Mount Sinai was blanketed in smoke, and the entire mountain trembled violently. They saw thunder and lightning and heard a blaring trumpet that continued to grow louder and louder. The Israelites kept their distance from the mountain, both out of fear and reverence.

Then God spoke to them, and they received the renowned Ten Commandments. The first words that God said were these,

"I am the Lord your God,

who brought you out of Egypt,

out of the land of slavery.

You shall have no other gods before me.

You shall not make for yourself an image in the form of
anything in heaven above or on the earth beneath or in
the waters below. You shall not bow down to them or
worship them; for I, the Lord your God, am a jealous
God, punishing the children for the sin of the parents to
the third and fourth generation of those who hate me,
but showing love to a thousand generations of those who
love me and keep my commandments." (Exodus 20:2-6)

The Lord continues with the remaining commandments. Afterward, the Israelites inform Moses that they do not want to hear

40

from God directly because they are terrified that they will die. They preferred to listen to the rest of His instruction indirectly through Moses. Moses attempts to reassure them that God was not trying to scare them but instead displaying His power and sovereignty as the one, true God so they would obey Him. Nonetheless, Moses continues to serve as an intermediary and receives the breadth of God's laws to share with the Israelites. The Israelites agree to the laws and commandments, saying, "Everything the Lord has said we will do." (Exodus 20:18 – 24:3)

If they had remained faithful to their word, I wouldn't be writing this chapter.

Maybe they had good intentions? I don't know. But what happens next serves as a great lesson and example for our journey.

Upon God's request, Moses ascended back up the mountain to receive the written instruction for His laws and commandments (Exodus 24:12-18). Scripture describes Moses' absence as 40 days and 40 nights, but to the Israelites, he was simply taking too long. They decided to approach his brother, Aaron, who had been left in charge. Notice Exodus 32:1-6:

When the people saw that Moses was so long in coming down from the mountain, they gathered around Aaron and said, "Come, make us gods who will go before us. As for this fellow Moses who brought us up out of Egypt, we don't know what has happened to him."

Aaron answered them, "Take off the gold earrings that your wives, your sons and your daughters are wearing, and bring them to me." So all the people took off their earrings and brought them to Aaron. He took what they

handed him and made it into an idol cast in the shape of
a calf, fashioning it with a tool. Then they said, "These
are your gods, Israel, who brought you up out of Egypt."

When Aaron saw this, he built an altar in front of the
calf and announced, "Tomorrow there will be a festival
to the Lord." So the next day the people rose early and
sacrificed burnt offerings and presented fellowship
offerings. Afterward, they sat down to eat and
drink and got up to indulge in revelry.

That was quick, right?

They had just seen a tremendous display of God's power and agreed to revere Him, comply with His commandments, and receive further instruction from Him through Moses. But when God didn't move according to their personal timeline, they decided to take matters into their own hands.

They had grown tired of waiting for Moses' return, and they were determined to make a god for themselves in whom they would place their trust. They were willing to mold and shape their possessions into an image that met their expectations, desires, and circumstances. And they celebrated their creation as the one that delivered them from their hardship.

That sounds a lot like the mother who gave me the questionable advice.

In her mind, her miracle babies were the outcome of the influence that she had in demanding that God provide her with children. She believed it was her own strength that delivered her from the hardship of infertility. She had grown tired of waiting and submitting her requests in prayer, so instead, she made demands and felt rewarded for her assertiveness.

Where I used to feel intimidated by her conviction, I now feel grateful that I don't share her perspective.

If someone serves a god that they can boss around—that's not a god, that's a genie. And it is a thinly veiled disguise of considering themselves as having god-like power.

When life doesn't go according to our expectations and plans, people will frequently comment that we have not received our desired outcome because we are not praying hard enough.

There is no "magic" number of prayers we can pray to promote our will. Pray fervently, pray incessantly, pray with a heart of gratitude, and make your requests known to the Lord, but never forget which one of you is the Creator and which one the created. Prayer is not a means of providing instruction to a hearing-impaired, impotent god that serves to fulfill our every desire. It's not a scheme to force His hand. Instead, it's a means of communion, communication, and glorifying the God whom we recognize as utterly stronger and more powerful than we could ever imagine or strive to be. It is a means of seeking His guidance, abiding in His presence, obtaining peace, expressing gratitude, sharing our emotions, fighting against adversity, and pleading for help for ourselves and on behalf of others. Prayer is an act of submission and strength. Our prayers are powerful—not because of our own strength, but because of the mightiness of the One to whom we are praying.

The following scripture keeps me encouraged and fortified when cynics try to convince me that a prolonged season of infertility is evidence that God has distanced himself from me and my prayers.

In 2 Corinthians 12, Paul writes about an affliction that has been given to him, which continually torments him. In verse 8, Paul conveys that he pleaded with the Lord three times for it to be removed. How did the Lord respond to Paul's prayer requests? Notice 2 Corinthians 12:9-10

> *But he said to me, "My grace is sufficient for you,*
> *for my power is made perfect in weakness."*
> *Therefore I will boast all the more gladly about my*
> *weaknesses, so that Christ's power may rest on me.*
> *That is why, for Christ's sake, I delight in weaknesses,*
> *in insults, in hardships, in persecutions, in difficulties.*
> *For when I am weak, then I am strong.*

If you're not familiar with Paul, he is a powerhouse of the Bible. He is credited with writing nearly half of the books of the New Testament. He was a devoted Jewish traditionalist who relentlessly persecuted followers of Christ until his own encounter with Jesus on the road to Damascus. His intensity in following Jewish laws and customs was then transformed into personal devotion to the teachings of Jesus. He dedicated his life to preaching and teaching the gospel, missionary work, planting churches, and extending the ministry to Gentiles.

If there was any man that had an intimate relationship with God, it was Paul. God used Paul's background, his mind, and his zeal to shape the early beginnings of Christianity.

But God did not remove Paul's affliction.

Bible scholars will debate the nature of Paul's affliction — whether it was physical, spiritual, emotional, etc. But the point remains that there was a personal matter that troubled Paul so much that he pleaded with God to take it away, and God did not do it. Yet God gave him an answer that many of us would struggle to accept. He said His grace was sufficient. His grace was going to be just as good (if not better) than removing his affliction altogether.

Why?

Because in our weaknesses, we find our true strength.

In our weakness, we can see the full extent of Christ's power.

What power have you witnessed *because of* infertility? What power have you observed in the midst of infertility? Not the power that came from you, but the power that came to you. If you haven't seen it yet, be sure that your emotions aren't clouding your perspective.

I would not be able to write this book without the power (strength) that continues to come to me. This topic is incredibly and emotionally hard, but the resources and opportunities that made it possible for this book to come to fruition was nothing short of strength from God. And the impact that these words may have just because of my silent womb is nothing short of amazing. I'm a young, Black American girl living in South Korea writing to you about the goodness of God BECAUSE of my weakness.

Isn't that something?

Our weaknesses do not exist because God has left us; our weaknesses are the best platform for people to see God through us. Don't be discouraged from believing that your prayers are not good enough, but be empowered to see that you have been given God's grace and God's strength in light of your weakness. If God used one of the most devoted men of the Bible to demonstrate power in weakness, what makes us believe that we do not have power in our weakness? What makes us believe we have to fashion for ourselves worthless trinkets and desires into idols? What we perceive as silence may actually be grace.

The Israelites were eager to make a god for themselves—not because they were in imminent danger or because they were starving or lacking basic necessities. All things considered, they were doing well. But they wanted a god because they were tired of waiting. They were tired of the silence. They wanted to be like everyone else who carried their "god" with them.

The golden calf that was made from their jewelry was not a coincidence. It was a reflection of the pervasive idolatry that existed around them and what they witnessed during their bondage in Egypt. They turned to idolatry because of what they saw. Even though God called them to be different and forbade them from making idols and bowing down to them, they did it anyway because of how they felt.

Whether we are tempted to look to ourselves for power or dabble in prevalent cultural and paganistic fertility rituals, we have to use every ounce of our strength to say no. We must abstain from it. We cannot let our feelings (whether from frustration, disappointment, or desire) cause us to participate in something that we know to be an enemy to our faith and our relationship with Christ.

I know how bad it hurts to see mothers with their children and wish it was you with your child. I know how bad it hurts when social media or community events make you feel excluded. I know the anxiety that arises when reflecting on the uncertainty and inequality of infertility outcomes. As it stands, the woman at the beginning of the chapter wears the crown of motherhood, and I still do not. But I no longer feel imprisoned by her perception of my weakness because I know that God's grace abounds (Romans 5:20). I know He uses our weakness (2 Corinthians 12:9). I know His silence is not His absence (Zephaniah 3:17 NASB). And I know we will always have a way to escape temptation (1 Corinthians 10:13).

So, when you're feeling crushed and weary, commit those truths to your heart and know that an extended season of waiting is not a sign of spiritual defeat and abandonment. Be cautious that you don't drift away from God. His grace is near and more powerful than you can imagine.

In Summary

- God gave the Israelites instruction to worship only him and to refrain from idolatry. The Israelites became indifferent to God's commandments when they grew impatient and uncertain about his timing. They created their own idol and began to worship it. We can be tempted to idolatry when we become frustrated and believe that God has distanced himself from us.

- There is power in our prayers, but when our afflictions remain in spite of our prayers, use it as an opportunity to discern how God could be using your weaknesses. Christ's power manifests in our weakest moments. Our strength comes from Christ, not of ourselves.

- We have been given God's grace. Whether or not we become parents, we have been given a gift that is abundant for our needs. Even when our situation continues to grieve us, the truth remains that God is with us. We each have a personal responsibility to ensure that our emotions do not cloud this perspective and tempt us into separation from God.

Chapter 5

Resistance

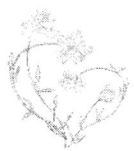

Shadrach, Meshach, and Abednego replied to him,
"King Nebuchadnezzar, we do not need to
defend ourselves before you in this matter."

Daniel 3:16

My husband, Richard, is incredible.
There's not much he wouldn't do for me. He's compassionate by nature, so his desire to serve comes naturally. He doesn't mind taking over my household tasks when I'm feeling sick or tired. He's easygoing and not one to ruminate over difficult decisions. He takes charge when he has to but gladly leaves the execution details to me. He's a man that seeks peace in his home.

I've hardly ever heard Richard raise his voice. He prefers to resolve conflict with thoughtful discussion and compromise. He chuckles at the famous marriage manifesto, "happy wife, happy life," totally convinced that there is a lot of truth behind those words.

Richard's desire to keep a happy home by ensuring my happiness comes a little too easy for him. He tries to keep a smile on my face, sometimes by his own volition and sometimes not. But I quickly and readily admit that there are many times when I am spoiled.

I've learned that I'm not alone. Apparently, in many marriage relationships, it's quite common for husbands to have a "fix it" approach when it comes to problems. Regardless of whether they're presented with a broken sink or a broken heart, they just want to know how they can fix it. That's certainly true in my marriage. While I am more into exploring root causes, connections, and details, my husband is totally solution-oriented. His laser-focused question is always, "What can I do to make this right?"

That works well for broken appliances, but not so much for infertility.

Our struggle through infertility turned what should have been romantic acts of intimacy into mechanically timed appointments. It turned special moments of togetherness into nightly syringe injections of astronomically priced medications. It transformed the art of conception from a private activity into an event where my husband waited across the room, watching a doctor perform some procedure. And it turned every negative pregnancy test into an emotional meltdown.

While I struggled with never-ending questions of "Why?" my husband only had one question: "What can I do to make this right?"

Richard, like many other men, hates feeling helpless. He has a heart that is drawn to making things better. If there is anything that really bothers him, it's to see someone suffering or hurting. He's the man who interrupted our anniversary photoshoot because he noticed a homeless guy that could use a few dollars. He's the man who drove an hour and a half in the middle of the night to meet a friend whose car broke down on the highway. He's the man who has dedicated the entirety of his adult life to serving in the military.

He's the man who would make an awesome father, if only he were given a chance.

There's a tremendous amount of guilt that I wrestle with as a barren wife. I know my medical circumstances are far beyond my control, but to see how my condition impacts my husband's opportunity to become a father is a difficult thing to witness on an ongoing basis. The guilt makes me so unhappy, and at times, even desperate.

While many Christian women dealing with infertility relate to the sadness, grief, and brokenness of Hannah, I am drawn to the stories of Sarah and Rachel. I wholeheartedly empathize with their feelings of desperation. Sarah saw that her window of fertility was closing, and Rachel couldn't stand feeling like a loser. They made decisions out of desperation, doing whatever they could to help their husband become a father. I'm so grateful that the Bible includes their stories because I know those feelings all too well. The pain and determination behind a decision made from desperation are undeniable.

In fertility desperation, I completely drained our financial resources to pursue medical treatments marketed as hope but more closely aligned with gambling. In fertility desperation, I continued to take medications and foreign supplements that created unnatural and dangerous side effects for my body. In fertility desperation, my husband and I have considered outrageous ideas that seemed palatable to our baby-hunger, only to realize the lunacy of such ideas once we became sober-minded. And in fertility desperation, we tried to "just adopt."

I am quite a force to be reckoned with when I am feeling hurt, guilty, and desperate. When I want my way, I can be very convincing—

let's be honest, intimidating—because I want to be right or happy. And many times (though not all the time) Richard complies. He stands alongside me, ready to support the approach that will result in a happy wife and a happy life.

That's what a loving husband should do, right?

Not always. But I am grateful that in my moments of pouting and conceitedness, I can instead seek God's gift of grace, repentance, and forgiveness.

This next lesson from the Israelites has proven beneficial to both Richard and myself as we learned to navigate the tough decisions and compromises that inevitably accompany an experience with infertility.

Insight from the Scriptures

In the last chapter, we discussed Exodus 32:1-6 and how the Israelites grew impatient in waiting for Moses' return and instead decided to make and worship a golden calf. I don't want to gloss over a critical part of this narrative, found in verses 3-5:

> *So all the people took off their earrings and brought*
> *them to Aaron. He took what they handed him and*
> *made it into an idol cast in the shape of a calf, fashioning*
> *it with a tool. Then they said, "These are your gods,*
> *Israel, who brought you up out of Egypt."*

> *When Aaron saw this, he built an altar in front*
> *of the calf and announced, "Tomorrow there*
> *will be a festival to the Lord."*

Notice the important character in this event—Aaron.

Aaron was Moses' brother, who had been temporarily left in charge while Moses was on Mount Sinai. Aaron was approached by a crowd of anxious Israelites who were eager to have a god in their midst. It was Aaron who suggested, received, and formed the jewelry into an idol. It was Aaron who attempted to justify their act by designating the idol worship as a festival to the Lord. Aaron made a compromise to appease an emotional crowd. He tried to take something unrighteous and turn it into something holy. He didn't initiate the idea, but he sure did have his hands in it, especially as a leader.

Happy Israelite, happy God?

Oh no, not hardly!

Because the Lord is omniscient and omnipresent, He knew what the Israelites had done. While the Lord was speaking with Moses, He tells him,

"Go down, because your people, whom you brought up out of Egypt, have become corrupt. They have been quick to turn away from what I commanded them and have made themselves an idol cast in the shape of a calf. They have bowed down to it and sacrificed to it and have said, 'These are your gods, Israel, who brought you up out of Egypt.'

"I have seen these people," the Lord said to Moses, "and they are a stiff-necked people. Now leave me alone so that my anger may burn against them and that I may destroy them. Then I will make you into a great nation."
(Exodus 32:7-10)

God was not happy. At all.

If you can't tell how furious God was by his description of the Israelites as "stiff-necked," His emotion described as burning anger, or His intent to destroy them, notice how He relates to them. He now calls them "your people, whom you brought out of Egypt." He was so enraged by their actions that He didn't want to associate with them.

The Israelites knew what they were not supposed to do, but they did it anyway. And their actions were shepherded and condoned by the one who had been left in charge—Aaron.

Upon Moses' plea for favor and leniency, and because of the Lord's great mercy, God relented in his anger. But when Moses returned and saw for himself the extent of their revelry and idolatry, he became livid. In his rage, he threw the two tablets of which God had inscribed the covenant law. He also destroyed the idol and made the Israelites drink its ashes (Exodus 32:11-16, 19-20).

Moses did not waste any time addressing his brother, whom he assumed had stronger leadership skills. He says to Aaron, "What did these people do to you, that you led them into such great sin?" (Exodus 32:21).

Moses not only wanted to know what happened, but he wanted to know what kind of actions/behavior/harm the Israelites had inflicted against Aaron to cause him to have such a lapse in judgment. You can see it in his question, "*What did these people do to you...?*"

We know that the Israelites didn't *do* anything to Aaron. We know that an aggravated crowd approached him, and he was likely feeling intimidated, but they never actually *did* anything to him.

Aaron cowered in his response to Moses. He said,

> *"Do not be angry, my lord"... "You know how prone these people are to evil. They said to me, 'Make us gods who will go before us. As for this fellow*

Moses who brought us up out of Egypt, we don't know
what has happened to him.' So I told them, 'Whoever has
any gold jewelry, take it off.' Then they gave me the gold,
and I threw it into the fire, and out came this calf!"
(Exodus 32:22-24)

Aaron completely shirked responsibility! He evaded accountability for his actions. Instead of owning up to feeling intimidated and making an unwise compromise, he says something like, "You know how these people are." And instead of accepting the blame for making the idol, he claims that he threw the jewelry into the fire (and somehow) a calf came out.

Really, Aaron? ... Really?

Yet, in the absurdity of his response, I still have great appreciation for how this narrative applies to our experience with infertility.

In trying to maintain the happiness of their household, spouses may find themselves making a compromise. Certain compromises are indeed healthy for resolving conflict, but we have to be on guard that our compromises do not conflict with what God has told us to do (or not to do).

It's not hard to sympathize with Aaron's position of feeling pressured and intimidated when faced with an emotionally-charged crowd, but we have to stand with the perspective that Moses had. Moses fully believed that his brother was a man of spiritual integrity and that only something grave could have caused Aaron to yield to such a bad idea.

Moses saw Aaron as an eloquent and persuasive public speaker. Aaron was the one who served as Moses' mouthpiece when Moses approached Pharaoh (Exodus 4:14-16, 7:1-2). That was undeniably an intimidating experience! But when left to serve as an independent leader, Aaron faltered.

In contrast, the Bible also gives us the gold standard for standing up to intimidation and refusing to compromise your beliefs. We find this in Daniel 3. In this chapter, King Nebuchadnezzar erects a towering golden image and makes a decree that all subjects, from every nation and tongue, must bow down and worship the image when they hear the music playing, or suffer the punishment of being thrown into a blazing furnace. But three Hebrew young men did not comply with this decree—Shadrach, Meshach, and Abednego. They refused to compromise their beliefs in the face of intimidation and power.

Notice their commitment and conviction when questioned (and intimidated) by King Nebuchadnezzar.

> *Shadrach, Meshach, and Abednego replied to him,*
> *"King Nebuchadnezzar, we do not need to defend*
> *ourselves before you in this matter. If we are thrown into*
> *the blazing furnace, the God we serve is able to deliver us*
> *from it, and he will deliver us from Your Majesty's hand.*
> ***But even if he does not**, we want you to know, Your*
> *Majesty, that we will not serve your gods or worship the*
> *image of gold you have set up." (Daniel 3:16-18)*

Wow.

They didn't attempt to debate the matter, nor was there any wavering in their mind. The young men were simply not going to do it. They didn't care how angry it would make the King, nor how much he could intimidate them. They had faith that God could save them from the furnace, but they were fully prepared for the outcome if He did not. That's how much they loved God. That's how much they were willing to keep His commandments without compromise.

That's a stark contrast from Aaron and the Israelites.

So the question is, where are we willing to draw the line in our journey? Where are we ready to take a stance in our desperation to resolve infertility?

There are many, many ways to try to "have a child;" some more innocent than others, but all options have consequences that must be assessed with a sober mind.

In total honesty, infertility-related discussions are the hardest conversations that my husband and I have had to deliberate. We have had to weigh all sorts of considerations—medical, financial, ethical, spiritual, moral, and personal. Those types of conversations would be hard for any couple, but when you do it within the highly emotional context of the desire to have children, it becomes incredibly daunting.

It's not lost on me the weight of infertility on the family dynamic. Not only does it present the obvious hurdle to expanding a family, but it creates a towering fear of how the inability to conceive a child will impact the marriage. Richard and I both have had to navigate years of insecure feelings, silent thoughts, and hard conversations about what would happen to our marriage if he never becomes a father, or I a mother. Yet even in the face of fear, we recognize that we're both called to maintain our commitment and spiritual integrity without compromise. You absolutely, positively cannot have infertility-related conversations with the singular agenda of doing whatever makes you (or your spouse) happy.

Each of us has a different threshold, and our access to social and economic resources are indisputably unequal. We have various limitations to the medical, financial, and personal opportunities to become a parent. But when it comes to weighing the moral, ethical, and spiritual consequences of different paths to parenthood, there is a question that we must consider. Take a moment to reflect on Romans 8:35:

Who shall separate us from the love of Christ?
Shall trouble or hardship or persecution or
famine or nakedness or danger or sword?

Have you ever thought about that question in the context of infertility? It's considerably hard.

Will a nagging spouse cause you to concede in your conviction?

Will a broken heart lead you to walk away from your faith?

Will a burning desire tempt you to compromise your relationship with Christ?

Romans 8:37 goes on to say, "*No, in all these things we are more than conquerors through him who loved us.*" Just like what we learned in the previous chapter, we are strong because of our weaknesses. We are strong because of the power that comes to us through Christ Jesus (2 Corinthians 12:9).

So, where have we, The Mitchells, learned to draw the line? As the head of our household, and after lots of hard lessons, my husband will readily tell you that he (now) ensures our infertility journey falls under the declaration of Joshua 24:15:

"... But as for me and my household,
we will serve the Lord."

We're being careful that our next step does not compromise our integrity or our values. We're being prayerful. We're taking our time. And we're watching and waiting.

On top of that, we're grieving and bonding. We're strengthening ourselves and each other. We're consoling one another.

And we both are standing firm in faith in the face of intimidation and temptation, regardless of whether it comes from our spouse, our internal frustrations, or pressure from outside of our marriage. We're not going to make a compromise to what we believe to be true.

Why? Because the best lesson that comes from Aaron and the Israelites is that Aaron had to stand accountable for his own role with the idolatrous act. It wasn't good enough for him to blame "those people," nor was it good enough for him to try to justify the wrong thing by dedicating it to God. If it had not been for God's mercy and Moses' intercessory prayer, Aaron would have paid for it with his life.

Richard and I want to become parents, but if desperation and intimidation lead either of us to do something that would anger God, it's not worth it. We each know we have to stand accountable for our actions, and we won't be able to justify a poor decision by using our spouse as an excuse. We will continue to rely on God's grace until we can receive His gift.

We strive to be like the three young men who made it out of Nebuchadnezzar's furnace unharmed, unsinged, and not smelling like smoke because they trusted God. What's more, an angel of the Lord was present with them in the fire.

Think about that.

In Summary

- ❀ Men and women often make compromises for the sake of keeping their spouse happy, but we have to be willing to stand firm in our conviction if a request compromises what God has instructed us to do (or not to do). This is especially hard when the request comes from a deeply emotional place, such as what happens with infertility.

● We have to take accountability for our actions and our role within the decision-making process. Our wrongdoing is not justified simply because it was done to appease someone or because it was ultimately dedicated to God. Having a calculated plan to sin is not reflective of the life that God has called us to live, and is abusive of his mercy.

● Do not allow feelings of desperation, intimidation, or temptation to convince you to do something unacceptable. When times get hard, lean on each other and seek the grace that God has given to us. We are more than conquerors because of the power that rests on us.

Chapter 6

Present

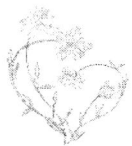

But if I go to the east, he is not there;
if I go to the west, I do not find him.
When he is at work in the north, I do not see him;
when he turns to the south, I catch no glimpse of him.
But he knows the way that I take;
when he has tested me, I will come forth as gold.

Job 23:8-10

I was devastated.

Heartbroken doesn't even begin to describe how I felt.

It's not like it was the first time I had ever received this kind of news, but for whatever reason, this time, it hit me pretty hard.

I was happy for her, but once the happiness subsided, I felt nothing but pure and utter devastation. I felt like my world had ended. I felt like I had no reason to smile ever again.

The more I scrolled on social media, the worse I felt. Every photo, every comment, every 'Like' felt like a cruel tease. But I was addicted to it. I couldn't stop. I wanted to see more, but I hated myself with each new image. I wanted to stop reading, but I was hypnotized by each post.

"Congratulations!"

"Oh my goodness, look at those cheeks! I'm so happy for you!"

"Your baby is so precious! What a beautiful gift from God!"

"You're so blessed!"

Tears had already started to well, but now I was fully weeping. My husband had already seen the pictures and had no words for me. He just put his arm around me in silence and kissed my forehead. He was sad about our situation, but mostly he was bothered that he didn't know how else to comfort me. We sat there quietly... staring at nothing... saying nothing, until he decided to give me a moment to myself. He kissed my forehead again, left the bedroom, and gently closed the door.

I cried into my pillow in a futile effort to muffle the sound of my sobbing, but it was no secret that I was in anguish. My eyes were swollen, my nose was running, and my spirit felt like it weighed a ton.

I was emotionally paralyzed. I didn't leave the room for hours. I had no appetite nor any desire to see anyone. I just cried... and cried, and cried, until my well of tears ran dry.

I realized why this particular baby announcement left me feeling so shattered. It was the fact that this child arrived in the most miraculous way I have ever heard. I was ecstatic for the parents, but this miracle left me with an unbearable question:

"Lord, why won't you do the same for me?"

Every time I started to feel like I had regained my composure, this question would run through my mind, and my heart would break all over again.

"Why, Lord? ... Why?"

I grabbed my prayer journal and started writing down each of my thoughts as a letter to God. It was the only way I could try to purge the feelings of misery and brokenness from my heart and mind. With each blank page, I poured out all of my hurt and despair.

Nearly each of my friends and family members has children. Many have never had to deal with infertility, and some have even become parents reluctantly. Most of the ones with prior infertility have ultimately become parents by childbirth or adoption, and the slight few that never became parents live with a pain so intense that they prefer not to speak about it.

And I understand their silence. They've stopped talking about their pain because no one has anything new to offer. No one knows what to say beyond, "I'm sorry," and maybe sit for a few moments before carrying on with their own life. I understand their silence because they've found it more useful to muffle their pain in an effort to rally the remainder of their strength to focus on the rest of life's challenges. But their pain continues to grow silently, often unnoticed and forgotten by others—the outsiders who feel too awkward and helpless because they don't know what else to do, effectively leaving the brokenhearted to manage the grief on their own. So broken ones don't speak about their pain, because they're doing everything in their power to keep from falling apart.

I reflected on my years of infertility and gazed at my emotional scars. It seemed like no matter how much I tried, how hard I prayed, how much I cried, how long I waited, nothing had moved God into blessing my path to parenthood. I felt dismayed and confused. If He planned to "give me hope and a future" and "the desires of my heart," why was I so unhappy? Why was everyone else receiving their heart's desire, but not me? I felt like a failure.

"Lord, what more do you want me to do?"

Insight from the Scriptures

If there is any part of the Israelites' journey that I want you to embrace, it's this segment right here. It's so important but so unassuming. If you're not careful, you might miss one of the greatest lessons we could possibly discover for our journey through any and every hardship.

Moses received meticulous instructions from the Lord about how to erect the tabernacle and how each of its furnishings and elements should be designed. The Lord provided the workers with an abundance of skills, abilities, and resources to get this assignment done. An incredible amount of precision and attention to detail went into the construction, furnishing, and operation of the tabernacle because it was where the glory and presence of the Lord would dwell. Once the tabernacle was completed, sacred procedures and laws established, and everyone organized into their roles and positions, the Israelites departed from Mount Sinai towards the promised land.

It had been two years, but just like when they left Egypt and were guided through the Red Sea, God's presence appeared to them as a pillar of cloud by day and a pillar of fire at night (Exodus 13:21-22).

Take a moment to reflect on Numbers 9:15-18, 21-23:

On the day the tabernacle, the tent of the covenant law, was set up, the cloud covered it. From evening till morning the cloud above the tabernacle looked like fire. That is how it continued to be; the cloud covered it, and at night it looked like fire. Whenever the cloud lifted from above the tent, the Israelites set out; wherever the cloud settled, the Israelites encamped. At the Lord's command the Israelites set out, and at his command they encamped. As long as the cloud stayed over the

tabernacle, they remained in camp. ... Whether the cloud
stayed over the tabernacle for two days or a month or a
year, the Israelites would remain in camp and not set out;
but when it lifted, they would set out. At the Lord's
command they encamped, and at the Lord's command
they set out. They obeyed the Lord's order, in accordance
with his command through Moses.

When God moved, they moved. When God stayed, they stayed. Yes, the obvious message from this passage is obedience and being attentive to the movement of God. But what stands out most to me, and what is most relatable to our experience with infertility, is when God did not move.

Verse 22 states that "Whether the cloud stayed over the tabernacle for two days or a month or a year, the Israelites would remain in camp and not set out; but when it lifted, they would set out." God didn't move, and sometimes he didn't move for an extended amount of time. And when he didn't move, the Israelites didn't move. They remained in their present location.

It's not necessarily the obedience that stands out to me; it's their position and the varying amounts of time that they spent in their location. The length of their journey was not solely based on their faith, their acts of worship, or their obedience, but also by the path and the duration of time that God spent moving. In His own divine wisdom, and for His own divine purposes, sometimes God moved, and sometimes He was stationary. We can contemplate and speculate the reasons behind His movement, but the fact is that He never provided an explanation. The best thing that the Israelites could do in those circumstances was to be obedient—and not just obedient about following Him, but about staying in their present location when God was motionless.

What do you do when God doesn't move?

Trust Him, yes. But we also have this amazing opportunity to communicate with Him in prayer. The truth is we might be using our prayers to ask Him why He is not moving, and if your journey has been anything like mine, He is not so responsive to that question. But fear not, you're in good company! He did not provide an explanation to the Israelites, either.

Nor did He provide an explanation to Job.

In the very first verse of the book of Job, we learn that he was "blameless and upright; he feared God and shunned evil" (Job 1:1). But as the narrative progresses, we witness Job losing his possessions, his children, his health, and the support of his wife and friends. Job was overwhelmed with misery and was struggling emotionally, physically, and spiritually. Like many of us, he struggled with understanding why he was experiencing such intense hardship and tragedy. He knew that God was good and that he had not done anything deserving of punishment. He couldn't reconcile "the why," and it troubled him.

Take a look at Job 23:3-7:

Even today my complaint is bitter;
his hand is heavy in spite of my groaning.
If only I knew where to find him;
if only I could go to his dwelling!
I would state my case before him
and fill my mouth with arguments.
I would find out what he would answer me,
and consider what he would say to me.
Would he vigorously oppose me?
No, he would not press charges against me.

Present

There the upright can establish
their innocence before him,
and there I would be delivered forever from my judge.

Job was desperate for just one conversation with the Lord so that he could understand the purpose of his suffering. His friends tried to convince him there must have been some grave sin he committed as a precursor to his situation, but Job was confident that he could defend himself against any accusation of wrongdoing. He was determined to find God and inquire about his affliction. He just needed a moment to plead his case. He just needed to know "Why."

If there is any question that has become the soundtrack of my infertility journey, it is "Why?". Like Job, I have internalized my adversity and examined myself to determine what I have done to deserve years of heartbreak and heartache. I have struggled to reconcile why my journey to parenthood has been longer and more difficult than others. And, similar to Job, I have had friends and family arrive at unhelpful and hurtful conclusions that further discouraged my understanding of God and His love.

The truth is that there will be times when our circumstances are directly the result of our own actions and decisions, but there will also be times when God is stationary, and it has absolutely nothing to do with what we have or have not done. Sometimes we "reap what we sow," but other times, God simply decides not to move. And He doesn't tell us why.

What has been hard for me is remembering that we are not all on the same journey. Even though we're invited to be encouraged by the experience of other infertile families, we have to remember that our paths may be similar, but they are not identical. I'm sure I'm not alone when I state that one of the worst parts about infertility is watching God move along someone else's path while He remains stationary in yours. Even the Bible captures this sentiment in the infertility stories of Hannah and Rachel as they respectively watched Peninnah and Leah become mothers. It's hard to watch someone receive your heart's desire, and it is difficult to balance your support for what God is doing in someone else's journey while mourning and wondering when He will move again in your story.

Yet, no matter how long God remains stationary, we must hold on to the truth that although He stops, He never leaves.

He never left the Israelites; His presence remained observably over the tabernacle. He never left Job; His eyes and ears were always attentive to him.

And He will never leave us.

We have this promise from Jesus when he declares in Matthew 28:20, "And surely I am with you always, to the very end of the age."

We have the presence of the Lord, and this presence makes all the difference. He is present on our journey, regardless of whether He has stopped or whether He is in motion. It is the presence of the Lord that we have to see as immeasurably more valuable than anything we could desire.

That's a hard truth. A very, very hard truth. But continue to bear with me.

Consider the fact that the Israelites were in the wilderness—a barren, unfavorable environment. They had everything they needed but didn't have everything they wanted. It was no secret they were tired of eating manna and living in the desert. They resented their journey. Their complaints were audible, and they were visibly weary. But the Lord was present with them.

In contrast, the Canaanites lived in the promised land—the fertile land "flowing with milk and honey," and the destination to where the

Israelites were traveling. The Canaanites enjoyed strength, power, and bountiful crops. But the Lord was not with them. They practiced idolatry and served many gods.

Ask yourself, who was blessed?

Were the Canaanites blessed because of what they had? Or were the Israelites blessed because of *Who* they had?

Your perspective on that question will make all the difference on your journey.

It's not the gifts (the blessings) that make you blessed; it's the One from whom those gifts were given. It's whether His presence is present. Romans 11:36 reminds us that

For from him and through him and for him are all things.

To <u>him</u> be the glory forever! Amen.

We place so much attention on "all things," that we often neglect to appreciate the One from whom it came. And, that One is the same One that is present when we are moving along our path, and still present when we are stationary. He doesn't become good once we receive whatever gift He has for us, but He always was and remains "good" during the entire journey.

We're not blessed at the moment we receive something; we're blessed when we abide with the One who does the blessing. It's not contingent upon our receipt of anything other than Him.

When you change your perspective from the gift to the Giver, you will realize that you are no less blessed than those who receive the gift. You will realize that you are no less blessed than those who have received the thing you have been praying for—your heart's desire.

Children are a blessing. They are a marvelous gift that comes directly from the Lord—a heritage and a reward, just as described in

Psalm 127. They are justifiably and rightfully something for which we should pray and grieve as we navigate through infertility. I am overjoyed when children are welcomed with every ounce of love they deserve. And we should remember that they are a blessing because of the One who formed them in the womb. They are a blessing because of that same One who is with us.

Everything we receive in this life would be insignificant if it were not for the One to whom we give our glory and praise. I wholeheartedly encourage you to read the book of Job in its entirety and see what Job couldn't see during his suffering. You will learn that his affliction had nothing to do with whether or not he was trying hard enough and nothing to do with proving his worth. His trial was a demonstration of whether his love for God was sincere or merely a result of everything he had received.

It's the same question that we face today, "Do we love God only because of what He has given us, or do we love God because of who He is?"

So many people have hardened their hearts or abandoned their faith because they have not been able to reconcile God's goodness with a particular void that exists in their life. Whether this void exists because of infertility, the loss of a loved one, or any other thing that their heart treasures, it's hard to say that "God is good" when you only seek to fill the void with what has been lost. It's hard to say that "God is good" when all you can see is your pain. But we have been invited and encouraged to fill that void with his presence. In Matthew 5:4, Jesus tells us, "Blessed are those who mourn, for they will be comforted."

Blessed.

We are blessed by His presence in our most profound hurt, even when we haven't received the fulfillment of our prayer request.

In my sorrow of seeing another child arrive that was not intended for me, I was still blessed. When God is stationary on my journey, I am still blessed. Even though He doesn't give me an explanation, I am blessed. Even if my story ends differently from how I have prayed, I am blessed. I have to stand firm against every disparaging thought that seeks to compare my circumstance to the gifts that God has given to other families because I know being blessed is not a competition but a description of the relationship I have with God.

Even though I have not received the blessing of children, I abide with the One from whom all blessings flow. In the depths of my tears, He is still present with me.

I am no less blessed.

In Summary

- As God guided the Israelites to the promised land, there were times when he was stationary. The Israelites were obedient and encamped when they saw that he stopped moving. Sometimes the Lord remained motionless for an extended period of time, and although He didn't provide the Israelites with an explanation, they remained obedient in following His movement.

- In the book of Job, we witness how Job endured hardship and affliction despite being a faithful servant of the Lord. His hardship was not a reflection of any wrongdoing, but a test of whether his faithfulness was motivated by his sincere love for God or a result of all the good things he had received.

- When we change our perspective and define "blessed" in terms of the Giver and not the gift, we realize that the greatest gift we could ever receive is the presence of the One who gives and not an item. We remain blessed when we continue to abide in the presence of the Lord. He blesses us with more than just things, but by filling our deepest void and supplying our deepest needs.

Chapter 7

Present, Still

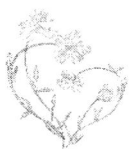

But Jesus replied, "My Father is always working, and so am I."

John 5:17 NLT

One day I received an unexpected message from the social media manager of a well-known health and wellness website. She had seen a comment I made on the topic of grieving and wanted to know the most helpful advice I had received while navigating a season of grief. Without hesitation, I remembered a quote that a dear friend shared with me when my father passed away. My friend had also lost a parent, and she encouraged me by saying, "Grief is not something you get over; it's something you get through. And you will get through it as many times as you need to." Because of this perspective, I have wholeheartedly become an advocate of the grieving process.

It takes courage and strength to be vulnerable enough to grieve, and it takes wisdom to recognize the need to grieve a loss. We commonly limit the grieving process to death, but grieving is indeed associated with different types of loss. We can grieve for more than just loss of life. We can experience a loss with our hopes, dreams, expectations, desires, security, or a change in circumstances. And yes, we can grieve the loss of our fertility.

I cherish the advice that "grief is not something you get over, but something you get through" because I have found it to be undeniably true. Whether the loss is an individual event (such as the death of my father) or recurs multiple times (such as the losses I have sustained on my infertility journey), the grief is not something you can simply push past. You must find a way to go through the process and heal through it, and this process does not occur overnight or with one attempt. Grief manages to return in waves and from triggers. And getting through it requires a level of strength and courage that you can only muster with support and experience.

And that's OK.

We were never created to get through life by ourselves, but the loneliness and emptiness created by loss can be so intense that we're tempted to dismiss how painful it can be. Sometimes we try to be self-reliant by withdrawing and convincing ourselves no one cares or understands, or we have to figure everything out on our own. As a result, we end up creating more problems than we solve. And whether it comes from pride or shame, we try to ignore the need to stop and grieve whatever ails us.

I understand the desperation that lures someone to try to numb the pain of loss. Two months after my father died, I pursued advanced fertility treatment. My father's death created a void in my family, and I was desperate to replace what had been lost. If I couldn't get my father back, I wanted to do everything I could to overcome my infertility. I tried to use hope and busyness to numb my pain. I kept a full calendar of medical appointments. I scoured online forums for treatment information, I monitored my diet, exercised, took a ton of medication and supplements, and prepared my mind and home for the child that I knew would arrive and exchange my emptiness for joy. The excessive financial investment I placed on my family, and the physical strain that I forced on my body, were irrelevant to my sole desire to feel whole again. This pace continued for several months until my stamina, money, and health declined.

So, I slowed, but I never stopped.

The next year, I pursued foster-care adoption with just as much intensity. I busied myself with books on trauma, attending conferences, watching webinars, studying child profiles, completing medical and social background investigations, and completing the required classroom training. But it led to the biggest heartbreak that I continue to shoulder because I was not emotionally prepared.

I never stopped to embrace the grieving process.

I wanted to keep going and push past all of my internal cries for help. I wanted to maintain my momentum in pursuing a child for our family, and I viewed my determination as fuel for endurance. But I couldn't ignore the fact that I was in the middle of an emotional breakdown that had gradually seeped into other areas of my life. Although I didn't want to face the truth, I reluctantly accepted I needed to pause my pursuit of family building options. As a result, all attempts down the different paths to parenthood came to a halt.

To create the space I needed to seek help and heal, I removed myself from several commitments and obligations. I allowed myself the freedom to acknowledge my losses: the loss of my father, the losses from years of unsuccessful fertility treatments, the growing loss of cohesion in my marriage, and the profound loss of a disrupted adoptive placement.

At that moment, I didn't need a child. I needed to heal.

I needed the opportunity to grieve.

Insight from the Scriptures

In the previous chapter, we learned there were times when the Lord was stationary as He led the Israelites to the promised land, and wherever He settled is where they would camp. Sometimes He was motionless for multiple days, and they remained encamped until He was ready to move again (Numbers 9:22-23).

In like manner, we will imitate their experience and camp with the understanding that sometimes God is stationary on our own journey. We previously learned even if God stops, He doesn't leave. But there is a second lesson we must embrace about God:

Even if the Lord stops moving, He doesn't stop working.

When we are stationary, God's presence and his pause allow us the opportunity to grieve, and we are given the comfort of grieving without grieving alone. The hard part, however, is believing when we stop to grieve, we are not forfeiting our hope and the opportunity to continue towards the ending God has prepared for us.

Yes, we can both grieve and hope simultaneously. Grieving is not a waste of time.

This fear is especially real for couples enduring infertility because of the constant pressure of racing against a clock. Whether it is the biological clock we hear ticking from a medical perspective, our own internal deadline for becoming a parent, pressure from family members, or our desire to maintain momentum with our peers, we become familiar with the phrase "time is of the essence." We are driven to keep moving.

But at what cost?

We have a choice to either pursue a path of self-determination and self-reliance or trust that God is still working even when our journey has come to a standstill. It may be hard to believe God can be present and stationary with us, yet simultaneously working and moving on a separate path that intersects with our journey. But that is precisely what He did with Naomi in the book of Ruth.

In Ruth 1:1-5, we learn that Naomi, her husband, and two sons lived in Bethlehem until they moved to Moab to escape a famine. While in Moab, Naomi's husband dies, and her two sons marry Moabite women: Orpah and Ruth. About ten years later, Naomi's sons also die, thus leaving her without a husband or her children.

When she learns the famine has ended in Bethlehem, she decides to return home. She urges her daughters-in-law to return to their homeland and re-marry so they will have a better life than what she anticipated for them in Bethlehem. Note Naomi's position in Ruth 1:11-13:

> *But Naomi said, "Return home, my daughters.*
> *Why would you come with me? Am I going to*
> *have any more sons who could become your husbands?*
> *Return home, my daughters; I am too old to have*
> *another husband. Even if I thought there was still*
> *hope for me—even if I had a husband tonight and then*
> *gave birth to sons—would you wait until they grew up?*
> *Would you remain unmarried for them? No, my*
> *daughters. It is more bitter for me than for you*
> *because the Lord's hand has turned against me!"*

She had reached a place where it seemed God had stopped moving. She had no hope and no means to create a life that would benefit her, Orpah, or Ruth. She didn't want them to endure the bitter fate of poverty and destitution that awaited her, and she encouraged them to pursue a different path. Both of her daughters-in-law loved her dearly, and although Orpah complied, Ruth insisted on staying with Naomi.

Naomi had Ruth's support, but she told the town to call her "Mara" because she felt that God had made her life bitter. In her heartbreak, she stated, "I went away full, but the Lord has brought me back empty...The Lord has afflicted me; the Almighty has brought misfortune upon me" (Ruth 1:21). Yet, as we continue to read the narrative, we learn that God had not stopped working. Naomi's story didn't end there amid her heartbreak, because things were happening in Ruth's story that would consequentially benefit Naomi too. Because of Ruth, Naomi was never hungry or abandoned. And by no coincidence, Ruth worked in the field of Boaz, a relative of Naomi's husband. Because of his kinship relation, he was able to redeem the property of her deceased husband and marry Ruth.

Through Ruth, Naomi did not have to succumb to the life of hunger and misery she anticipated. And, she even received the unexpected pleasure of living her elder years loving on her new legal son, Obed, who would ultimately become the grandfather of David and an ancestor to the Messiah (Ruth 4:17).

It's inconceivable, literally.

God may have been stationary (with Naomi), but He was still working (through Ruth). And when He was ready to move again with Naomi, He brought her to the intersection of the work He had done through her daughter-in-law, a place that she could not have fathomed during her heartbreak. He brought her to a joy that she thought she would never see, nor would have been able to create herself.

That's great! But what does that have to do with our infertility journey?

In the depth of our loss, and when it appears that God has stopped moving, our minds can paint a grim picture of the life we imagine to be awaiting us. In the infertility community, we continuously talk about the brokenness and heartache we experience, but we rarely discuss the fears we wrestle with on our journey:

- The fear that we will never become a parent

- The fear that we will never be happy if we don't become a parent

- The fear that we're missing out on one of the greatest of life's experiences

- The fear of experiencing a miscarriage or pregnancy loss

- The fear that our marriage won't survive if our spouse does not become a parent

- The fear that physical intimacy has lost its value

- The fear that we will end fertility treatments prematurely

- The fear of failure

- The fear of shame and stigma

- The fear that we're being punished or deemed unworthy

- The fear that God is not listening

- The fear that God does not care (or even worse, is not real)

I know this list is not exhaustive, but it is certainly exhausting. I admit my mind and heart have drifted towards many of the items on this list, and I'm saddened to think about the men and women who have succumbed to some of these fears.

These fears paint a hopeless picture of what life would be like if we're unable to conquer infertility, and it drives us to keep striving towards the ending we're hoping for—even if our bodies, finances, loved ones, mind, and spirit tell us to pause. We want to push past it. We want to get over it.

But the fear resulting from untended grief is not something that we can simply get over; it's something we must go through. I have found that when you stop and recognize a circumstance as a loss and grieve through it, it prepares us for whatever next step God has arranged.

Imagine if Naomi just tried to push past Ruth's determination to join her. Imagine Naomi being so consumed with fear about Ruth's life in Bethlehem that she continued to encourage Ruth to return to Moab. But Naomi did not give in to the fearful mental picture in her mind. Instead, she relented.

There's no one way to grieve a loss, and everyone's season of grieving will look different. But there is an undeniable truth that the healthy way to grieve is by not going through it alone.

God loves each of us more than we could ever understand. And even in her heartbreak and bitterness, even despite her resolve to see God as the one who afflicted her and brought misfortune upon her, God loved Naomi enough to ensure she would not grieve her loss alone. But Naomi had to stop and let go of her fears in order to receive the comfort God wanted to provide through Ruth.

So, stop and think.

Who are you pushing away? What coping tools, opportunities, and resources are you declining because you want to push past your loss and give in to your fears?

What is God currently trying to do for you in the place where He has stopped in your journey?

Jesus tells us that the greatest commandment is to "Love the Lord your God with all your heart and with all your soul and with all your mind" (Matthew 22:37). But when fear consumes our heart, soul, and mind, it's hard to be faithful to this commandment. We can try to push past it, but we have to be honest with ourselves. Do we end up giving Him a superficial love—a love that tries to hide how we *really* feel inside; prayers that are rote, shallow, and ineffective?

God wants every part of us. The good, bad, broken, hurting, fearful, devastated, and hopeless. He wants it all. Just because He has stopped moving, doesn't mean He has left. Just because He has stopped moving, doesn't mean He has stopped working, both *for* you and *with* you.

He provided Naomi with Ruth. And in His love, He also gives us support and resources.

Richard and I have worked very hard to build a strong marriage, and Richard is a fantastic support and companion for this difficult journey through infertility. But because God loves both of us, Richard is not the only resource He has given to me.

God has given me professional counseling, peer support groups, fellow warriors against infertility that I have not met by coincidence, and spiritual sisters who understand the strength that comes from being vulnerable and talking about their pain. He has given me stronger prayers, better Bible study, and the tools and resources to grieve and grow, right in my present location. He has given me the ability to love Him authentically and embrace our highest commandment.

We don't have to deny our heartbreak or our troubled mind; instead, we can ask Him to provide healing, comfort, and hope through support systems, just as He did for Naomi.

God is present in the moment-by-moment struggles and day-to-day challenges. He is not so far that we don't have access to the opportunities, resources, and relationships that He makes available to us in our losses. We can truly rely on Him.

When we see ourselves as 'no less blessed' because of this access, it gives clarity to how suffering produces perseverance, how perseverance produces character, and how character produces hope (Romans 5:3).

It was Naomi's character that motivated Ruth to stay alongside her. It was Naomi's character that enabled Ruth to trust her, love her, and establish the setting for which both of their blessings manifested.

Hardship reveals our character, and the decisions we make during a season of adversity reflect our values. The opportunity to stop, grieve, and utilize the support and resources God makes available to us is not a sign of weakness or forfeiture, but an invitation to strengthen ourselves and be encouraged by His love during a difficult journey.

It is indeed the path to the hope and future He has prepared for us. It is the encouragement to trust that He has not stopped working on our behalf; that even when He has not moved, He is present, still.

In Summary

- 🌼 Grieving is an essential tool for the healing process. We commonly associate grief with death, but grieving involves different kinds of loss. Infertility is a type of loss we can (and should) grieve. If we feel that God has stopped moving on our journey to parenthood, it may be an invitation to stop and grieve our losses and use the resources He makes available to us.

❀ Even though it seems God has stopped moving, it does not mean He has stopped working. It may be that He has brought us to a place in our journey where it intersects with someone else's path. It is in our best interest to trust Him and to not "push past" the spot where He has placed us. Instead, we can use it as an opportunity to rest and heal.

❀ It is hard to love the Lord with ALL of our heart, soul, and mind when our mind is consumed with fear. Fear keeps us from welcoming the good things that God is working to provide to us. There are many fears in the journey through infertility, and it takes strength and courage to not give in to those fears.

Chapter 8

Unfulfilled

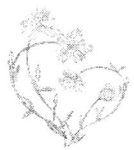

My sacrifice is a humble spirit, O God;
you will not reject a humble and repentant heart.

Psalm 51:17 GNT

Twelve years ago, I stood outside of an ice cream shop and watched a glossy black Ford Mustang pull into the parking lot. I listened to the engine calm from a roar into a purr as the driver downshifted and glided the coupe into a vacant spot. The engine silenced, and the driver stepped out of the car, dressed in a dark blue jumpsuit and aviator shades. He walked over to me, and confidently introduced himself, and 16 months later, that suave stranger became my husband, Richard.

And Rochelle, the smooth 2003 Centennial Edition Ford Mustang, was his baby.

Rochelle received all the love and attention a man could give his beloved car. She was never dirty, always shiny, and Richard was incredibly picky about where he parked. He drove her everywhere, and I enjoyed being a giddy passenger, happy to be chauffeured around town in a sleek ride. Richard and Rochelle welcomed me into their precious relationship until my husband and I discussed whether a two-door sports car was compatible with our desire to have a 'real' baby.

I distinctly remember Richard's very masculine, yet tender, sadness as he exchanged the icon of his bachelorhood for the practicality of a mid-sized family SUV. But that sadness has now gravitated towards me. Had I known we would spend ten years without the need for a family-sized vehicle, we might have been able to embrace Rochelle a little bit longer. I miss the fun the Mustang brought to our lives.

If I'm being honest, infertility is no longer the daily 'doom and gloom' experience it once was. I've learned to appreciate the energy, resources, and opportunities Richard and I experience as a couple without children. We're able to invest in our marriage, fully address our individual needs, and serve others. Our lifestyle positions us to continue doing the things we enjoyed in the early years of our marriage (albeit without Rochelle), while still having freedom from the responsibility of parenting.

We have a decent life.

But there's a quote attributed to Theodore Roosevelt that says, "Comparison is the thief of joy." And man, how true that is!

Life is good, but then something will trigger and remind me of how parenthood is an experience I have to watch from the sidelines. Sometimes it's an unexpected baby announcement, a photo or video featuring an adorable kid, the arrival of child-centric holidays and events, or simply watching the children of my friends and family reach new milestones. All the good that Richard and I have, and everything that I am grateful for, gets eclipsed and caught up in an emotional whirlwind of sorrow, vulnerability, and longing. I'm reminded of how many times we have been unsuccessful at trying to create those experiences for ourselves, and I start feeling like a failure. I begin to feel empty and hollow, and the fullness of the word "barren" descends upon me. Barren starts to describe more than just my silent womb; it feels like a part of my identity. I begin to question the depth of my happiness and gratitude, wondering if it's just a façade for deeper questions I can't answer, like: Why can't I be a mother? Why can't I gift the privilege of fatherhood to my amazing husband?

It's all I see, and all I want.

It's that 'one thing' we don't have.

If there were a shared experience in infertility and childlessness, I would bet it's the feeling of exclusion and heartbreak. Anyone who struggles with infertility and childlessness knows how it feels to be "the one who can't" when everyone else can, or the one who doesn't have what everyone else has. We each know how terrible it feels when desire goes unfulfilled.

There is nothing wrong with wanting to be a parent; it's an innocent desire. However, it's the emotional response from an unfulfilled desire where we have to be careful. We have to be cautious that our longing does not birth bitterness and anger and become an insidious seed that pollutes our attitude, perspective, or behavior.

I'll be the first to admit that this is hard. Comparison has, at times, been the thief of my joy. I've spent many days irritated, frustrated, and sometimes downright jealous I don't have a beautiful child to raise. I ache for the pride, joy, and challenge of watching my child blossom. But alas, we're still just a family of two. I don't have cute photos and videos to share, and in many scenarios, I feel entirely left out. You don't realize how many conversations are about children until you don't have one to discuss.

I've had many bitter moments that lingered into bitter days, and bitter days that extended into gloomy months. But sour thoughts, left to fester, never lead to pleasant outcomes. And this is a vital lesson and direct warning from the story of the Israelites.

Insight from the Scriptures

I would be remiss in discussing the trek of the Israelites without mentioning the bitter complaining that persisted throughout their journey. Many of the Israelites did not make it to the fringe of the promised land because of how much they angered the Lord with their attitude and audacity. Because they were determined to remain disrespectful, their journey was cut short; and for some of them, so were their lives.

There are several examples of their complaining we could examine, but the most common complaint was about the provision—manna. What was once a miracle and a blessing had now become meaningless and detestable to them. Beginning in Exodus 16:14-16, manna appears on the desert ground each day. These thin flakes were to be gathered, ground into flour, and made into bread for the Israelites to eat. The Israelites ate manna every day, and by the time we reach Numbers 11, they had been eating manna for over two years. Notice their posture in Numbers 11:4-6 (HCSB):

> *Contemptible people among them had a strong craving for other food. The Israelites cried again and said, "Who will feed us meat? We remember the free fish we ate in Egypt, along with the cucumbers, melons, leeks, onions,*

and garlic. But now our appetite is gone;
there's nothing to look at but this manna!"

Sure, seasoned fish and vegetables are delicious! It's an innocent desire to want that kind of meal. But the problem was not that they craved different food; it was that they were harboring a bitter and ungrateful attitude. Their unfulfilled desire for the food they left behind in Egypt enticed them to narrowly focus on the one thing they did not have, instead of appreciating all that they had received.

They longed for the food they ate while in Egypt but failed to balance that longing with remembrance of what accompanied such tasty food. They had good food but lived as slaves. They had good food but spent 400 years being beaten and oppressed and pleading to the Lord for their deliverance. And now, they were free from slavery, being formed into God's chosen nation, and being led to fertile land, all in exchange for temporarily enduring a monotonous menu. Yet to them, it wasn't worth the cost.

In addition, the "contemptible people" (also called "the rabble" or "the mixed multitude" in alternate Bible translations) were the ones who instigated the grumbling in this particular example. The mixed multitude included the crowd of Egyptians and other foreigners that accompanied Israel out of Egypt[2]. They were not committed to the Lord with the same dedication He required Israel to have, yet their attitude had a distinct impact on the Israelites. Their influence, along with Israel's own bitter mindset, lured the Israelites to join alongside their criticisms.

The collective wailing and complaining of the Israelites and the multitude were so inescapable that it stressed Moses. He asked the Lord,

---

[2] Tyndale House Publishers. Study note on Numbers 11:4, in *The Life Application Study Bible: New International Version* (Carol Stream, IL, 2007), 208.

"Why have you brought this trouble on your servant?
What have I done to displease you that you put the
burden of all these people on me? Did I conceive all
these people? Did I give them birth? Why do you tell me
to carry them in my arms, as a nurse carries an infant,
to the land you promised on oath to their ancestors?
Where can I get meat for all these people? They keep
wailing to me, 'Give us meat to eat!' I cannot carry all
these people by myself; the burden is too heavy for me.
If this is how you are going to treat me, please go ahead
and kill me--if I have found favor in your eyes--and
do not let me face my own ruin" (Numbers 11:11-15).

Moses had the same repetitious diet as the rest of the Israelites, but he was more concerned with his obligation and responsibility as a leader. Moses wasn't so focused on what they did not have as much as he was eager to get to wherever God was leading them. But their attitude, and their complaining, was affecting his leadership ability and making his life miserable. Although he shared their struggle, he didn't share their perspective. He, too, was frustrated, but the instigators didn't influence him. His focus was elsewhere.

Ask yourself, where is your focus?

I'll admit, I have to make a very intentional effort to ensure my focus does not rest on the "one thing" that Richard and I do not have. I'm not saying that I never think about it, or that it doesn't affect me, but that I have to be deliberate in preventing bitter thoughts from getting comfortable, growing roots, and tainting my attitude and behavior.

You may be familiar with a popular illustration that describes how thoughts and feelings affect your attitude, beliefs, and, ultimately, your behavior and lifestyle. The model demonstrates how change becomes a little more difficult at each new level. Changing a lifestyle is much more difficult without changing the underlying behavior and belief system. And changing a belief is much more difficult without first changing the underlying attitude and feelings. When we allow bitter feelings to find a comfortable place to grow, they become rooted and established as bad attitudes, or worse, a cynical way of life.

A recent series of disappointments on our path to parenthood affected my attitude. After I had received several setbacks and denials from adoption agencies, I found it very difficult to congratulate my friends on welcoming the new additions to their families. It seemed like I couldn't catch a break, and I started to feel incredibly bitter about my situation and jealous over their happiness. I had to be intentional about spending some time alone to grieve and pray and uproot those feelings before they had an opportunity to settle.

One of my favorite scriptures to pray in those moments is Psalm 51:10, where David writes, "Create in me a pure heart, O God, and renew a steadfast spirit within me." David was repentant and remorseful because he had committed adultery with Bathsheba, and he knew this sin would get in the way of his relationship with God. He didn't want to live a life apart from God, and he tried to uproot anything that would cause further separation and distance between the two of them. David, like the Israelites (and even us with infertility), was enticed to focus on the *one thing* he didn't have, and his emotional response fueled the decision to engage in unwise behavior.

Desire can be a tricky emotion, and we have to be careful about the voices that influence our attitude and behavior in response to our desires. Whether it is our own internal voice or an external grumbling, we have to be mindful of whether this voice shifts our perspective away from all that God has provided and all that He is trying to do in us, for us, and through us.

Just like the Israelites, we don't walk through adversity alone. There are people who may share our physical struggle, but not our spiritual commitment. They travel alongside us, just as the mixed multitude journeyed with the Israelites, enduring the same heartbreak and challenges but not the same beliefs. Collectively, we may vent and groan about our hunger pains because we can empathize and identify with each other. But the Israelites took their focus off of God, and their perspective for all that He was doing for them became skewed. What may have been acceptable for their neighbor did not align with their unique identity as God's chosen people. God was merciful to both the Israelites and the multitude, but as the nation who had been called to serve the Lord, the Israelites had to be careful not to become bitter in their attitude and relationship with Him. We have to do the same thing.

I always reflect on this when I participate in online support forums about infertility. While there is undeniable comfort and relief in speaking with other people who understand the trials, heartache, and frustration of infertility, I have to be cautious about how much I am being influenced or affected by the complaining of others. Many conversations in these forums focus only on the "one thing" we do not have and are not inclined to offer healing or perspective on everything else we have received. No, we should not deny our brokenness, but we can't live there either. We stumble in our faith when we envelop ourselves in hurt and bitterness instead of surrounding ourselves with people who can be both empathetic and encouraging. For this reason, I have learned to limit the amount of time I spend on infertility forums if it becomes evident that a particular group provides negligible therapeutic value and does not attempt to balance heartbreak with prayer and thanksgiving.

It is incredibly vital for us to seek voices of gratitude during our journey—voices that can be extremely sensitive to our hurt but still guide us to return our gaze towards the many things we do have while waiting for the one thing we don't have. It's good for our healing and our relationship with the Lord and with others. I did not fail to notice how much the bitterness and complaining of the Israelites affected Moses. It troubled him and burdened him because he personally had no means to alleviate their frustration. Does that sound familiar? Could that be happening in your relationship with your spouse?

In his love, God has provided me with a wonderful husband. However, Richard is not the only resource and support that God has provided because there is only so much my husband can personally do. The burden of infertility is too much for either of us to bear, and it would not be fair if I expected Richard to do what he has no means to do. But what we have done, which the Israelites failed to do, is to be the voice of encouragement for each other. We listen, we empathize, we are very transparent about our hurt and frustration, but we also try to keep a broad perspective. We don't want to fall into the trap of becoming too narrowly focused on the "one thing" we don't have.

Infertility still hurts immensely, but we are intentional about constantly shifting our focus to being grateful for God's provision and continuing to make our requests known in prayer. When we broadened our perspective, we recognized a child is one of the many representations of God's love, but it is not the *only* way He shows love. That's the unshakeable truth that took us many years to accept.

A child is not the only way that God demonstrates His love for us. And Rich and I have shifted our prayers from not just praying for our child to also praying for all of the children who have touched our lives, and releasing any bitterness or hurt from not being able to call these children our own.

It has given us a better perspective on God. Just because we have not been successful in growing our family does not mean He has not heard our prayers. Just because it hurts to see another family welcome a child does not mean He does not care about our pain. And just because something may trigger our tears, does not mean He is indifferent to our brokenness.

God is with us, and He is constantly blessing and demonstrating His love for us. We just have to be intentional about shifting our focus and taking a second look.

In Summary

- Focusing on "the one thing" you do not have can divert your perspective from appreciating the many things you do have. It can be detrimental to your faith and a barrier in your relationship with God.

- Our desire may be innocent, but we have to be cautious about the attitudes and behaviors that result from unfulfilled desires. If we allow bitter attitudes to grow, they can develop into unhealthy mindsets, actions, and lifestyles.

- We have to be mindful of how the complaining of others influences our own perspective. We should not deny our pain, but we have to find healthy, therapeutic environments that promote healing instead of constant venting. And, we must be intentional about creating a healthy environment in our relationship with our spouse.

Chapter 9

Crossroads

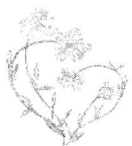

Each of you should use whatever gift
you have received to serve others,
as faithful stewards of God's grace in its various forms.

1 Peter 4:10

Author Note: *This chapter is difficult for me. In all honesty, I didn't want to write it. It was so emotionally challenging that I seriously considered giving up on this book altogether. For several months, I was paralyzed between wanting to complete this manuscript while also trying to avoid this particular topic. It's the one part of my infertility story that is still very tender, but I knew I could not write about infertility without discussing it. My challenge was knowing that this is a very delicate subject with a wide variety of passionate opinions. I was intimidated by the judgment and* *criticism I might receive from sharing my experience. It was a struggle to find a way to navigate these multiple layers of sensitivity, and it just seemed easier to give up and stop writing completely. Nevertheless, I persisted because I hated the idea of leaving this work unfinished; but mostly, I persisted because I knew there would be one person who would have loved to read this book once I found the courage to get through this chapter. But I would like to emphasize that there is no right answer on this subject, as there are many different experiences and perspectives.*

Everyone who experiences infertility arrives at the same crossroads. Regardless of your circumstances or the specifics of your diagnosis, if you stay on the journey long enough, the path will lead to the intersection of these five words: "Why don't you just adopt?"

I don't remember the first time it was said to me, whether it was a question from someone else's curiosity or my own internal thoughts, but I know it soon became an undercurrent to my infertility experience. The years of negative pregnancy test results; the times my husband and I lamented over the cost of another fertility treatment; the prayers that seemed to go unheard and unanswered; the jealous tears from watching other families welcome a child into their lives— left me in a numb silence with one question, "Why don't you just adopt?"

Just adopt.

Simply adopt, and all of this heartache goes away.

It's selfish of you not to consider the many children who eagerly await a loving home.

Just adopt!

In its simplicity, adoption connects a child with a family. These are just a few of the ways that adoption can occur:

- A family may contact a private adoption agency and use its resources to locate an expectant mother who is considering an adoption plan for her child.

- An expectant mother may arrange the adoption placement of her child with someone whom she has privately identified.

- A family may pursue an international adoption of a child residing in a foreign country.

- A couple may adopt an embryo using advanced fertility technology.

- An extended family member may adopt a child via kinship adoption.

- A step-parent may formally adopt his step-child.

- Or, a child in the custody of a child welfare organization may be placed with a family for foster-care with the goal of adoption.

I have participated in three different adoption opportunities. While I continue to see the beauty and promise of adoption, I also know that there can be a lot of pain when an adoption arrangement does not proceed in the way you had hoped. And it hurts all the more when uninformed bystanders continue to shout, "just adopt!"

In one scenario, a family friend contacted me and informed me that her daughter was expecting a child and considering an adoption plan. After writing a heartfelt letter to her daughter and speaking with her on the phone, she agreed to place the child with me. I researched and prepared the legal requirements, then eagerly converted a spare bedroom into a nursery and purchased every baby item I could find. When the child was born, the mother contacted me, and I arrived at the hospital to welcome the beautiful baby girl. A few days later, a third-party informed me the mother decided not to continue with the adoption plan and did not desire any future contact from me. While I wholly and genuinely respected her decision, I was devastated nonetheless. I was a complete emotional wreck as I tried to locate the receipts to return some of the baby items to the store while donating the rest to charity.

In another scenario, my husband and I decided to pursue adoption through a private agency. We were astounded by the cost of private adoption (tens of thousands of dollars more than fertility treatment), but we resolved that it would give us the best opportunity to become parents. We made a plan to liquidate all of our assets, empty our retirement savings, and apply for a substantial personal loan. In our preparation to interview adoption agencies, we educated ourselves about what to look for in a reputable organization. The more we researched, and the more interviews we conducted, the more conflicted we became. There were many, many adoption agencies using unethical practices—from manipulation and coercion of expectant mothers, to emotionally and financially baiting prospective adoptive families, to downright child trafficking. Not to mention, we became acutely aware of the racial bias in private adoption. The adoption cost for children of African, Hispanic, and Asian heritage was significantly less than the adoption cost for children of Caucasian descent. Babies were essentially a commodity—their value being influenced by the economic forces of supply and demand created by the adoption market. None of it is a secret, but much of it continues to be overlooked because of the emotional desperation of families seeking to welcome a child into their arms. Richard and I could have easily turned a blind eye to the red flags and disingenuously selected one of the many popular agencies that confidently assured us we would be successful using their services. But when we stopped and prayed about it, the answer was clear. Private adoption would absolutely allow us to become parents if we were willing to surrender the money and overlook questionable practices. We admitted to ourselves we were eager to become parents, but we were not desperate. Neither were we willing to be ignorant and inconsiderate of the impact of the adoption triad—the triangular relationship depicting the needs and sacrifices of each constituent in an adoption: the adoptive parents, the biological parents, and the child. Coupled with the challenge of being stationed overseas, we also had limited options in ethical agencies that were willing to work with us. There was no way we would agree to make a financial transaction on the sole basis of our emotions that would eclipse the voice of birth parents and adoptees and perpetuate the practice of a loosely-regulated industry. So, despite our heartbreak, we decided not to pursue private adoption at that time.

But our most poignant adoption experience occurred long before we even considered private adoption.

In the United States, children who have been abused, neglected, or lacking proper supervision by their birth families are removed from their homes and placed in the custody of a child welfare agency. Depending on the circumstances, these children are placed with a foster family while their birth family seeks resources and support to equip themselves for the child's return home or placement with a relative. Alternatively, the parent's rights may be legally terminated, and the child becomes available for adoption. A child whose parents had their legal rights terminated may wait several years for an adoptive family, and, as the child ages, adoptive families become less and less likely to pursue an older child. Unfortunately, these children may reach the age of adulthood without ever being adopted. Without a doubt, older children in the foster care system are the children most in need of an adoptive family. With this in mind, Richard and I became foster parents with the hopes of adopting an older child.

The foster care system is hard. There are limited resources and support networks, the social workers are overwhelmed, the children are doing their best to navigate through trauma, and foster parents face challenges atypical and unknown to parents with biological children. It can be a roller coaster, but foster parents will readily tell you that it is one of the most challenging yet rewarding experiences of their life. They have the rare perspective of being able to witness the growth and healing of a child that has progressed from hurting to thriving, from hopeless to hopeful, and from distrusting to loving.

But depending on the depth of trauma that a child has experienced, things may get worse before they get better. The child that Richard and I welcomed into our life came from a terrible history of severe abuse and abandonment. And although his siblings had all been adopted, he had been waiting for several years for his own "forever family." I remember being assured that my love, prayers, and determination would be enough to withstand the challenge of being his foster mother and, ultimately, his adoptive mom. But navigating through severe child trauma, a reticent welfare system, and a home environment that was steadily declining in safety and security was an overwhelming experience for me as a first-time parent. The hardest decision I have ever, ever had to make was to terminate our adoption plan for this child. There is unequivocally no greater sadness than telling a child in foster care you will not be his forever family, and watching his hopes dissipate behind a protective wall of rejection, self-reliance, and defeat. I felt like a monster and a failure. My own guilt and shame from that moment linger to this day, even despite having the confidence that we made the right decision.

When people say "just adopt," it implies a thoughtless, impulsive action—a straightforward problem-solution relationship with infertility and a disregard for any difficulties it may involve. But the decision to pursue adoption cannot merely be an emotional response.

Let's continue to take a look at the Israelites.

Insight from the Scriptures

In Numbers 13, the Israelites reach the southern perimeter of the promised land. The Lord instructs Moses to send 12 men to scout the land and validate its abundance. After 40 days, the men return and give a good report of the land's provision, but warn about the formidable enemies that reside there. Of the twelve scouts, ten promoted a bad report and incited fear amongst the Israelites—convincing them the enemies were indomitable giants that could not be defeated. Only two scouts, Caleb and Joshua, were confident that the Lord would bring victory to the Israelites. But the negative report of the ten scouts left the Israelites feeling distraught. They cried,

> *"If only we had died in Egypt! Or in this wilderness! Why is the Lord bringing us to this land only to let us fall by the sword? Our wives and children will be taken as plunder. Wouldn't it be better for us to go back to Egypt?" And they said to each other, "We should choose a leader and go back to Egypt" (Numbers 14:2b-4).*

Caleb and Joshua continued to try and convince the Israelites to have faith in the Lord, and said,

> *"The land we passed through and explored is exceedingly good. If the Lord is pleased with us, he will lead us into that land, a land flowing with milk and honey, and will give it to us. Only do not rebel against the Lord. And do not be afraid of the people of the land, because we will*

devour them. Their protection is gone, but the Lord is with us. Do not be afraid of them" (Numbers 14:7b-9).

But the Israelites remained paralyzed by fear and refused to be encouraged, and even considered stoning Caleb and Joshua to death! They continued their manner of grumbling and complaining, and it proved to be their ultimate demise. Instead of entering the promised land, the Lord declared that they would continue to wander in the wilderness until their deaths, and only their children would have the privilege of entering the land they rejected. When they heard this news, they were grieved and mourned all night. But the next morning, the Israelites were disobedient and crossed into the promised land anyway, against Moses' objection and without the presence of the Lord. They were attacked and defeated by the enemy and pushed back down the hill to their original camp (Numbers 14:26-45).

I struggled to write this chapter because I know there are challenges in pursuing adoption, and adoption is not always the easy, idyllic experience it is often portrayed to be. But I am incredibly careful when speaking about it because I never want to deter someone from pursuing an adoption opportunity. I never want to be the reason a child does not receive a loving and supportive home. Unlike the ten scouts who surveyed the promised land, I do not desire to incite fear and dissuade someone from trusting God. Instead, I aspire to be like Joshua and Caleb, who were very forthcoming and honest about the challenge that awaited the Israelites, but also very confident that it would be the Lord who would help them through it.

In the land of adoption, there are formidable giants. Just as the Israelites had to confront the enemy if they wanted to enjoy the promised land, prospective adoptive families will encounter challenges if they are going to experience everything that adoption has to offer. Some parents will contend with raising a child with varying levels of trauma; others will continually seek a delicate balance to incorporate the child's birth family; some will navigate the cultural and ethnic complexities of transracial adoption; and still, others will wrestle with the comments, perceptions, and insecurities that they are not a "real" mother or father. Certainly, there are additional challenges. None of these are small hurdles, for sure, but neither are they too lofty for God.

The need for adoptive families is substantial, and there is no question why the general public assumes that persons who want a child but struggle to conceive should readily welcome one of the many children waiting for a family. But instead of feeling pressured to "just adopt," each person should give very thoughtful, prayerful consideration to the opportunity and their readiness to adopt.

The biggest misconception about adoption is that it is a "cure" or fix to infertility. No, adoption does not cure infertility, but it is instead a path to parenthood. Infertility is one of the many routes that may lead to this path, but the pathway does not discriminate the fertile from the infertile. God calls, invites, and leads people to adoption— and this invitation is not exclusive to (nor specifically for) infertile families. There is a lot of synchronizing that occurs to bring an adoption to fruition, and, without a doubt, there is more to consider than the functionality of someone's womb when assessing the suitability of an adoption placement. Adoption specialists will readily admit that particular adoption scenarios welcome experienced parents or established families with children. And, there is an emotional preparedness prospective adoptive families must maintain that can be hindered if they have not adequately grieved their infertility-related losses.

Trying to seize the promised land without sincere regard for where God was leading did not fare well for the Israelites, and will not fare well for us, either. Our infertility journey should never be the sole focus of adoption, and being motivated to soothe our grief with adoption is a considerably selfish decision. Each person, irrespective of their fertility, should evaluate their emotional readiness and spiritual preparedness to pursue adoption as a path to parenthood. Thoughtlessly rushing into adoption out of emotional impetus is careless and has the potential to create additional problems for an innocent child, yourself, or an already fragile adoption system. Prospective adoptive families have the greatest influence in promoting ethical and culturally competent adoptions when they stop to assess themselves, their environment, and their underlying motivation to adopt.

But that is not to say that infertile couples should ignore the significant needs of the adoption community. The land of adoption, just like the promised land, is "exceedingly good." Those who are led to adoption must calm their fears as they trust God to help them slay the giants of the land, while those who have not been called to adopt but are sensitive to its challenges must find or create ways to use their resources and networks to help support the adoption community.

There will always be a need for both adoptive families and allies of adoption and family stabilization.

The scripture at James 1:27 is frequently cited as the rallying call to adoption. It states, "Religion that God our Father accepts as pure and faultless is this: to look after orphans and widows in their distress and to keep oneself from being polluted by the world." But limiting this scripture to an adoption action plan is a very narrow perspective. Instead, it calls us to serve others—specifically, those who are disadvantaged and powerless, such as orphans and widows, and to remain spiritually chaste. The opportunity to serve the less fortunate has no limits or bounds; and when we consider serving children, it includes adoption as one of many possibilities.

Undoubtedly, the most pressing need for children is a loving family and a healthy home. Yet good homes and strong families do not thrive without a supportive community. That's why we should not shy away from recognizing and discussing the challenges that are present in the foster care and adoption community.

When we provide support to families, we ultimately support the child. Foster and adoptive parents face many of the same problems traditional parents encounter, but they also have very unique challenges they cannot traverse by themselves. Some individuals serve as respite providers; ministries provide meals and supplies for foster families; organizations teach transracial adoptive families the critical importance of cultural competence and sensitivity; workshops provide continuing education for adoptive families beyond the adoption process; agencies work to make ethical adoption opportunities accessible to waiting families; and a myriad of other creative and supportive activities.

Not to mention, several individuals and organizations work with underserved communities to address the underlying challenges contributing to the abuse, neglect, and abandonment of children. Their goal is to mitigate the removal of children from their primary homes in the first place. And still, additional individuals and organizations seek to support expectant families by locating the resources they need to parent their child, recognizing that many expectant mothers and fathers would not place their child for adoption if they felt confident that they could suitably provide for the child's needs.

While there is no denying there are children who need adoptive families, there is also no denying that people who serve in supportive positions and share their God-given gifts and talents are just as crucial to the wellbeing and self-esteem of disadvantaged children. We need people to serve in both roles; children need both parents and allies in the community.

But the greatest lesson from this account of the Israelites is the reminder that our attitude is the most significant determinant in where our faith leads us. The first-generation Israelites were so close, yet so far. They were positioned just a few feet away from their new home—the land they were desperate to enter—but they couldn't get past their fear. Even though they had plenty of recent memories of God's protection, provision, mercy, and presence, it was still not enough to surmount the worst images of their imagination.

Some couples desperately want to become parents but are afraid of pursuing adoption. They fear what they have heard, what they have experienced, or what they believe in terms of the legitimacy of becoming a family via adoption. Although fear has the goal of protecting us from harm, it can also be incredibly limiting. It can keep us from participating in an experience that will favorably change our lives and the lives of others.

I have no doubt some couples remain childless because they reached the path of adoption, and like the Israelites, they trembled in fear, afraid of the giants that resided in the land. And, like the first generation of Israelites, they live the remainder of their days in despair, rejecting the abundance that awaited them.

But it does not have to be that way.

The best thing we can do during our infertility journey is to remain attuned to God's voice, guidance, and intention for our lives, and any direction about how we can use our gifts to help others. If we are called to the path of adoption, we must remain ready to listen, receive, and trust God despite our fears. Those who choose the path of adoption must walk with the understanding that their infertility journey was integral, but not superior, to the needs of everyone else that inevitably becomes involved in their decision. And, that God saw something in them, beyond their childbearing capability, that was crucial to his plan to expand their family.

We cannot be like the Israelites and make a purely emotional decision. We can't simply surrender to the masses that shout, "Just adopt!", and in our presumption, rush into a delicate environment without prayerful consideration. Instead, we have to listen to the Spirit that assesses our spiritual readiness and emotional preparedness to receive a uniquely curated blessing, and like all situations, continue to trust that if God leads us to the door of adoption, he will remain with us no matter the outcome.

In Summary

- We cannot "just adopt" merely because we have challenges with our fertility. The decision to pursue adoption requires thoughtful and sober consideration. We have to be aware of the unique challenges of adoption and respect the needs of everyone who inevitably becomes involved in the adoption triad.

- Adoption is not a cure to infertility; it is an opportunity to become a parent. And, there is a significant need for adoptive families, including those who have parenting experience and established families with children.

- Everyone is not called to adopt, but the adoption community is in desperate need of both adoptive families and adoption allies. If you are led to adopt, you must calm your fears and trust God to help overcome the challenges that are involved in adoption. If you are not called to adopt but are sensitive to the needs of the adoption community, find or create ways to use your talent, resources, and support networks to benefit the children and families awaiting adoption.

Chapter 10

Pathways

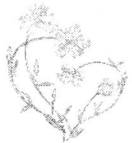

As for the seed that fell among thorns, these are the ones who, when they have heard, go on their way and are choked with worries, riches, and pleasures of life, and produce no mature fruit. But the seed in the good ground--these are the ones who, having heard the word with an honest and good heart, hold on to it and by enduring, bear fruit.

Luke 8:14-15 (HCSB)

"Guess what? I got my orders. We're going to South Korea." Of all the things my husband has ever said to me, this one had to be the most shocking. I barely allowed his words to sink in because I refused to believe him. He had to be joking.

"What? You're kidding, right?"

"No, I'm serious. Seoul, South Korea."

I honestly don't remember the rest of that phone call, but I do remember being at work when I received it. I abruptly told my manager I needed to go home, and out of concern, he asked if I was okay. In between tears, I managed to say to him, "We're moving to South Korea."

South Korea.

I didn't even know where it was. I knew it was somewhere in Asia, probably near Japan, likely close to China. I knew there had been a lot in the news about North Korea, so that explained this unanticipated assignment. But, wow... South Korea?

South Korea.

Every time I said it, the words triggered a new wave of tears and disbelief. It wasn't fair. It just wasn't fair.

After nearly a decade of searching, stressing, and trailing behind my husband's military career, I had finally found a good job—*a really good job*. And, we had just purchased a home. It seemed like we were finally generating enough stability to put down roots and settle into a normal life. For once, I could actually build a meaningful career instead of a string of random jobs. We could even reconsider fertility treatments now that we had become a dual-income household. But that was before the phone call. That was before the Navy decided we needed to move to South Korea.

It took a while for me to embrace the idea of moving to Korea. Once the initial feelings of shock and disbelief subsided, I felt bitter and angry. For months, I couldn't let go of how unfair this disruption felt to my hopes and dreams. Sure, we had moved before, but neither of us ever considered that we would take an overseas assignment. We didn't ask for it, and honestly, we didn't want it. But it didn't matter. We had a non-negotiable directive to move to Seoul.

While friends and colleagues were excited about my relocation to Asia, I was angry about what I was losing. I sincerely loved my job, and it had been an incredible blessing when I received it. It was a brand-new position that was created for me, a position that served as a testament to how much I impressed the company during my graduate internship. It was an introduction to a career for which I had not been qualified to apply, with access to invaluable mentors. That job provided me with my first taste of genuine financial stability and career development. Life was starting to feel good (for the most part). But now everything was being taken away. I'd likely spend the next few years underemployed if not unemployed altogether. How could God allow that? Why would he do that to me?

The only answer that gave me a sense of peace was to believe God had something waiting for me in Korea that was greater than what I was losing. It was the only way I could come to terms with leaving my job, my home, my country, my comfort zone, and all of my hopes and plans.

By the time we arrived in Seoul, I had already researched various organizations where I could volunteer and make community connections. I was determined to locate whatever it was that God had waiting for me—that thing that was so important that he would disrupt my life and bring me to the other side of the world. I buried myself in volunteerism, supporting charitable organizations, and networking with expatriate women from across the globe. My efforts ultimately led me to manage a visitation program with a local orphanage. My role was to help relaunch an opportunity for volunteers to hold and play with babies who were waiting to be adopted. But, until the group had enough volunteers to be self-sustainable, I would have to attend the weekly visitation with the infants.

Nothing compares to the peculiar feeling of walking into a room of children who do not have dedicated parents to care for them. It's indescribable. It's heartbreaking, for sure, but it's also perplexing. Your mind swirls with all kinds of questions: How can there be so many children without a home? What's his story? What's going to happen to her? And so forth. There is more uncertainty than answers, more sadness than hope.

Each week I caught the bus from my apartment to visit the babies for a three-hour shift. I played with them, fed them, and held them—trying to provide the warmth and love they deserved while at the same time ignoring my own emptiness and brokenness. I created a routine of using my bus ride to mentally disengage from my infertility-related emotions so I could be somewhat numb while visiting the children. Then, I would use the return bus ride to allow my heart and thoughts to wander with the freedom to feel sad and grieve.

It didn't take long for this mental routine to fracture. During each visit, I played with different babies—not wanting either of us to attach emotionally. But on one particular visit, I happened to pick up a small six-month-old baby boy who simply refused to allow me to let go of him. If I tried to put him down, he would wail, fuss, and disturb the nearby sleeping babies. But as long as I held him, he was wholly content. I sat in a rocking chair and rocked him gently, hoping that he would join his adorable friends in gentle slumber, but he had no intention of going to sleep. He just wanted to enjoy the moment of being held.

I couldn't help but reflect on how precious yet horrible that moment felt. He and I were suspended in a time where we met each other's deepest needs. He wanted a mother to hold him, and I wanted to be a mother. If given the chance, I would have gladly carried him out the door and returned to my apartment, ready for us to begin a new life together. But what kept us from formally uniting was not necessarily our differences in culture or the stark contrast of my skin color. It was not my language or background, nor my ability to champion his emotional, social, cultural, physical, educational, and psychological needs. No, none of those things mattered. It was money. I simply did not have the money to pursue private adoption for him (or any child for that matter). And it angered me that money was the horrible barrier between this precious child receiving a family and me becoming a mother.

So, I held this tiny baby for my entire shift. I let him enjoy every second of our silent rocking, and I stared into his innocent eyes for as long as my heart would allow it. He nestled himself into the crook of my arm and never made a sound. Even when it was time for me to leave, he remained silent as I returned him to his crib.

I walked to the bus stop in tears and decided I could no longer participate in the program. It was too emotionally difficult to be with orphaned children whom I would never have the opportunity to welcome into my family, yet simultaneously wrestle with the pain of infertility and the unfulfilled desire to become a mother.

Shortly after I left the orphanage program, I received motherhood announcements from two of my closest friends; and one friend inadvertently gave her baby the same name that Richard and I had been saving for years with the hope that it would, one day, be the name of our child. This series of back-to-back disappointments felt like a cruel tease. My spirit was crushed, and as a result, I withdrew into an extended season of loneliness, depression, and grief.

It wasn't fair. It just wasn't fair.

Insight from the Scriptures

He finally reached his breaking point. For years, Moses had endured their whining, complaining and grumbling about how they wish they had died in bondage, how they wanted another leader to guide them back to Egypt, how tired they were of eating manna, and so forth. He had interceded for them on countless occasions, pleading on their behalf before the Lord and asking the Lord to have mercy on the Israelites for their rebelliousness and ungratefulness. But this time, Moses lost his temper and went too far.

In this account, the Israelites antagonize Moses (again) because there is no water to drink. He was feeling frustrated and pestered. Note what happens in Numbers 20:6-12 :

Moses and Aaron went from the assembly to the entrance to the tent of meeting and fell facedown, and the glory of the Lord appeared to them. The Lord said to Moses, "Take the staff, and you and your brother Aaron gather the assembly together. Speak to that rock before their eyes and it will pour out its water. You will bring water out of the rock for the community so they and their livestock can drink."

So Moses took the staff from the Lord's presence, just as he commanded him. He and Aaron gathered the assembly together in front of the rock and Moses said to them, "Listen, you rebels, must we bring you water out of this rock?" Then Moses raised his arm and struck the rock twice with his staff. Water gushed out, and the community and their livestock drank.

But the Lord said to Moses and Aaron, "Because you did not trust in me enough to honor me as holy in the sight of the Israelites, you will not bring this community into the land I give them."

He was disqualified. Can you believe it?

Despite his faithfulness during the entire journey, this was a costly mistake for Moses. He let his irritation with the Israelites get in the way of obeying the Lord's command, and instead of speaking to the rock, he hit the rock twice and took credit for the miracle that ensued. It was a grave error, especially for someone with the responsibility of serving as a leader and role model for the nation of Israel. And for that, he was now forbidden from entering into the promised land.

Was the judgment a little too unfair? That depends on your perspective.

Without a doubt, Moses had to be held accountable for his actions, and the significance of his error necessitated a significant consequence. But we cannot be quick to say, "Moses lost everything." He would indeed miss out on a treasured opportunity, but not the opportunity of a lifetime. He was still a leader, still loved by God. He would continue to shepherd the Israelites and prepare his successor, Joshua, to be the one to lead the second generation into the promised land.

Moses could have easily become discouraged and even slipped into a deep depression or lashed out at the Israelites in anger. Hearing he would never enter the promised land had to be devastating, and knowing he would die in the wilderness could have convinced him there was nothing worth striving towards. He could have abandoned the Israelites and let them fend for themselves. What did it matter? It's not like it would make a difference, would it?

But that's not who he was.

He continued to hold his position with honor until it was time to commission Joshua as the new leader. He ensured the Levitical priests had appropriate records, and he taught the Israelites a new song to remind them of their mistakes and motivate them to rely on God. He remained faithful, and the Lord rewarded him with a panoramic view of the promised land just before Moses took his last breath.

Even though he never experienced it for himself, even though he only got to witness the promised land from the sidelines, Moses was no less blessed than the ones who received the treasured opportunity to cross into Canaan.

Does that sound familiar?

Infertility can be devastating. It feels like a miserable spectator sport – one where you know you possess every talent and qualification to participate, but for some reason, your opportunity (your blessing) is either delayed or declined. But Moses never saw himself as "less blessed" when he was barred from the promised land. And apparently, neither did God or the nation of Israel.

Israel revered Moses, and the Jews continued to respect him for his substantial role in delivering their ancestors from slavery and serving as the prophet through whom God established the law. Moses' reputation was far from insignificant, as evidenced by the directive in Hebrews 3:1-6 that we live under today:

... fix your thoughts on Jesus, whom we acknowledge as our apostle and high priest. He was faithful to the one who appointed him, just as Moses was faithful in all God's house. Jesus has been found worthy of greater honor than Moses, just as the builder of a house has greater honor than the house itself. For every house is built by someone, but God is the builder of everything. "Moses was faithful as a servant in all God's house," bearing witness to what would be spoken by God in the future. But Christ is faithful as the Son over God's house. And we are his house, if indeed we hold firmly to our confidence and the hope in which we glory.

Moses was not less noteworthy because he didn't reach a cherished destination. And it is the same for our own identity. While there is no shame in hoping and praying for our heart's desire, we have to hold on to this one steadfast truth that remains evident in the story of the Israelites, the example of Moses, and every other character record in the Bible: *our relationship with God is not so much about what we receive, but about who we become.*

Who are we going to become in light of our journey?

It wasn't where the Israelites were going that was important; it was who they were becoming.

Who have you become during your journey? Someone attentive to the movement of God? Someone who rests when God stops? Someone who can both receive and be a resource? Someone who believes that what awaits is superior to your fears? Someone who can stand firm in faith even when walking an undesirable path? Someone who can still pray and praise while in pain? Someone who can unequivocally say that God is their first love?

If our journey is only about the destination, then the Bible would have come to a close once Joshua led the Israelites across the Jordan River. But God was trying to do more than simply deliver the Israelites from bondage to freedom. He was developing them into a nation. He was setting them apart from people who had lost their way and turned their hearts from serving Him. His primary concern was with who they would become.

There is no doubt that the God of Israel has the same concern for us today. He is concerned with who we become amid our hardship, and that identity is much deeper than we could imagine.

As much as I want to continue to believe conquering infertility is about becoming a parent, I don't. I know if my personal journey weren't about infertility, there would have been some other adversity. Truly there is not a single person alive unscathed by pain and heartbreak, holding on to desperate hopes and prayers for fulfillment. I think about that every time I consider that within walking distance from the fertility clinic of my hometown, there is both a children's hospital and a general hospital. In each building, men and women are praying and asking God to heal their family. And a few blocks further are income-challenged neighborhoods where families are praying to make ends meet. And even here in Korea, the tiny 6-month-old baby boy that refused to let me put him down was praying in his own way that his deepest needs would be met.

The only distinction between our adversities is who we become in the process and how we respond to fear.

There are countless infertility books and resources that will encourage you to keep praying, keep waiting, and keep holding on until you receive what it is you are praying for, and I won't detract from that message. Instead, I give you the same advice that Moses left to the Israelites: "Be strong and courageous. Do not be afraid or terrified ... for the Lord your God goes with you; he will never leave you nor forsake you" (Deuteronomy 31:6). It's the same insight that David (another of God's beloved leaders) provided to his son Solomon in 1 Chronicles 28:20, saying, "Be strong and of good courage ... do not fear nor be dismayed, for the LORD God--my God--will be with you. He will not leave you nor forsake you..." (NKJV). And it is the same comfort that Jesus himself gives to us in John 14:27, saying, "Peace I leave with you; my peace I give you. I do not give to you as the world gives. Do not let your hearts be troubled and do not be afraid."

If the three greatest leaders in the Bible share the same wisdom, it has to apply to infertility too. We cannot be afraid of how God uses this hardship to guide us to becoming the man or woman he desires us to be.

Being in Korea has allowed me to reflect upon my journey through infertility. No, I have not become a mother, but I have become wiser. I have not succumbed to disappointment and bitterness, but I continue to mature emotionally and spiritually instead. And I no longer fear the outcome of my infertility journey, but I have come to a new perspective on what it really means to be blessed.

In God's great love, Moses went from feeling intimidated by a speech impediment to becoming a powerful orator and eminent leader of a nation. And though Moses never set foot into the promised land, Joshua had the privilege of having him as a mentor and role model.

Even if my husband and I never experience the miracle pregnancy of the infertile women of the Bible, or set foot into the land of parenthood, it would be an honor to have the opportunity to be able to instill wisdom and be an example of faith for the next generation of leaders the way that Moses did for Joshua. No, it's not the same as parenting or being able to enjoy everything that comes along with having a child, but it was an extraordinary distinction that even Joshua's own parents could not provide to him.

And no, it does not diminish the sadness or grief. Perhaps even Moses saw the land of promise with tears in his eyes, wishing he could personally experience it, but he knew God had neither left him nor forsaken him. He knew God loved him, and he knew even though he may have been brokenhearted, he had not "lost everything."

So, as I sit here in Seoul with just a few months left before we return to America, I have a better appreciation of what God was doing in bringing me here. He is not simply concerned with my womb, my career, or my family finances. He's not merely an answering service to my prayer requests. No, He's concerned about all of me, and all of who I am. He's developing me.

Being in Korea provided a unique opportunity for me to form relationships with people who understood my deepest hurts, visit places that challenged my Americanized view of the world, and spend extensive time studying God's Word. He's shaping me into the woman He needs me to be for whatever plan He has that awaits me. I have no idea what that means in terms of whether or not my husband and I become parents, but I do know that I can see there is nothing that God wouldn't do to demonstrate His love for me and connect me with resources to help on the path to the woman I will become—bearing fruit, whether or not that means bearing children.

Even though God knew Moses would never enter the promised land, he still saw that Moses had an incredible gift that would be instrumental to His plan. We, too, have a unique gift that God can use if we are willing to muster the courage to be the person He desires us to be and keep walking on the path that leads to His plan. It's the plan that gives us "hope and a future," an inconceivable plan without comparison, on a path that is *no less blessed.*

In Summary

- Moses did not become less notable because he did not enter the promised land. He was important because of the leader that he had become and the relationship with God that he modeled for the Israelites. Similarly, we are not "less blessed" because we are challenged with infertility. Our identity and purpose and God's love for us are not diminished if we do not carry the title of mother or father.

- Our relationship with God is more about who we become on the journey than what we receive. The person we become prepares us for the destination where God leads us.

❋ Don't be afraid of what God is trying to do with you, for you, and through you in this season of hardship. Our experience will indeed change us, and it can reveal the incredible gift we each have that God will use for His plan.

Afterword

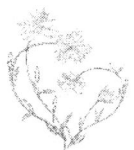

This is not a book that ends with the triumphant story of miracle motherhood. Nor is it a story that ends with the acceptance of a childless life. It is merely the last chapter of a story still in progress.

I honestly don't know what the next chapter will look like, but what I do know is that I completed this book with an incredible amount of peace.

I will be OK.

I no longer fear whether my story will end with the manifestation of what people have come to expect from an infertility story. I no longer fear whether pregnancy is a symbol of God's approval of me and His acceptance of my prayers. I no longer fear this time and opportunity that he has provided to me to grieve my losses. I no longer fear joining a community of men and women who long to become parents but have been rerouted to an alternative path. I'm not afraid of whatever outcome awaits me. I am not afraid because I know that whatever may come, it will be OK.

When I think of where I am in my infertility journey, I know, undoubtedly, that I have "let go." To be clear, "letting go" is not a declaration that I have given up; neither is it a statement that I have walked away from God. On the contrary, it means I have released my vision and my hopes and expectations to God for Him to use for what He deems to be "good." I want Him to use His creativity to bring about that uniquely customized ending that is waiting for my husband and me.

No, letting go is not giving up. Letting go is trusting that all will be well. Letting go is walking into a place of fear and pain while still believing that God is good. It is trusting that He is stronger than the hurt I am feeling and compassionate enough to lead me out of depression and despair. Letting go is believing when I feel like I am sitting on the sidelines watching women enjoy the crown of motherhood, the Lord reminds me that I, too, have my own crown —I am a beloved daughter of the King of Kings. Letting go is walking away from the unhealthy mindset of comparing my life to someone else's life, and instead, resisting the urge to compete. Letting go is genuinely believing that what's for me is for me. Letting go is opening my eyes to behold the gifts and opportunities that have been placed in front of me right here, and right now.

But I have been on this journey long enough to watch other men and women "let go" in a different context. They have let go of believing life can be good even when it looks different than their hopes and prayers. They have let go of marriages because it did not produce a child. They have let go of the promise for "the peace that surpasses all understanding" (Philippians 4:7) and allowed anger and bitterness to fill the void of unfulfilled desire, silent prayers, and a broken heart. They have let go of their faith in God, and have let go of any belief in His presence or His love for them. Their context of "letting go" is simply walking away.

For better or worse, pain entices us to let go. The deep, emotional pain of infertility convinces us to seek ways to defend ourselves from suffering additional pain. We numb ourselves to child-centric experiences and environments and from interactions that remind us of our deferred dreams and secret tears. And, if left unrestrained, we numb ourselves to the need for a relationship with God. I know I did. I couldn't reconcile myself to love someone who possessed the effortless power to wipe away my pain. I didn't understand why I should incline my heart to someone who seemed not to incline His ear to my prayers. But everything changed the moment I opened my eyes and took a look around.

Have you ever just stopped and took a silent moment to look around? Not to observe what you have, but to appreciate what has been created. We don't live in a simple, monochromatic world with just one of anything. There is not merely one color; one texture, one pattern, or one living creature. Instead, we live in a world of a myriad of colors, textures, patterns, plants, animals, and more! An immensely creative God formed a world of unlimited design. And located somewhere within that design is your life and your story. If God can use his creativity to design what you can see, imagine His potential with what you have not yet seen.

And still, recognize that His creativity is not confined to the limits of our imagination. That awareness led me to a place of understanding that the biggest tragedy of infertility is not the inability to have a child. No, the biggest tragedy of infertility is that we use our hopes and expectations to limit our perspective of God's creativity and what he can do with our story. But we have to let go of our vision and give His vision a chance. We have to trust that our pain does not go unnoticed. We have to believe we are not "less blessed" than those who have received our heart's desire.

So, I let go.

And, my husband has let go too.

And with deep appreciation, we now hold on to what we have already received as we wait in expectation of the creativity of God. At this moment, we have each other, we have a new perspective on trust and faith, and we have valuable experience from a journey we never wanted to endure, but that has prepared us to connect with and comfort others. We walk with purpose and intention, knowing this experience has not been without merit or reason. We walk with love and confidence, knowing we are blessed, not because of a parenthood status but because of the presence of the God we serve.

I know everyone will not welcome this perspective. And, not everyone will understand you can feel both joy and pain simultaneously. But as anyone who has had to live with grief and loss will tell you, that is exactly the required skill to keep moving forward. It takes courage and strength to resist the temptation to numb yourself from emotional pain. It takes faith and endurance to withstand waves of grief, knowing you must allocate the space and time to heal and find a supportive community. And it takes an all-knowing, all-powerful, compassionate, and creative God to guide you through the wilderness of infertility to your promised land.

In the final days of writing this book, I struggled with making sure I said the right things—making sure I addressed the voices and experiences of an audience that often feels ignored and disregarded. I wanted to make sure that something in this book resonated with every man and woman dealing with infertility. I tried to represent infertile families of color; I tried to address both men and women; and I tried to view infertility beyond my modernized, American lens through which I see the world. I tried to take an omniscient view of infertility because I wanted each person to know they are seen, and they are loved. I genuinely wanted each reader to believe they are not "less blessed." But the peace I now embrace was not from trying to be the voice of every circumstance, but in being a voice that directs readers to the true omniscient, omnipotent, and omnipresent God that hears and sees their situation; and demonstrating faithfulness in summoning the courage to share my story.

As this book comes to a close, I pray that you welcome a new perspective as you continue on your journey. I pray you find ways to honor your experience, that you continue to build a thriving relationship with your spouse and connect with a community that provides genuine empathy and support. I pray that any tender and broken places in your relationship with Christ find healing. I pray that your void is filled, and that you do not let go and walk away. I pray that you receive peace and joy even amid your pain. And I pray, above all, you never forget or cease to believe that we worship a God that loves us more than we could ever know.

This last verse is a scripture that I treasure, and it has become the theme of my infertility journey on both good days and bad days. I pray that it gives you comfort as you continue to trek toward the place God is guiding you.

Though the fig tree does not bud
and there are no grapes on the vines,
though the olive crop fails
and the fields produce no food,
though there are no sheep in the pen
and no cattle in the stalls,
yet I will rejoice in the Lord,
I will be joyful in God my Savior.

Habakkuk 3:17-18

Acknowledgments

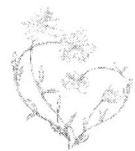

I honestly can't believe I've reached this section of the book. Even though it's the last thing I'm writing, it has not been the last thing on my mind. At every stage of writing this book, I have stopped to reflect in gratitude for the people and resources that came together to make this possible. From the friend who encouraged me to stop thinking it was such a "crazy idea" to write a book, to the proofreader who gave this manuscript a final look before publication, and everyone in between, I just want to say THANK YOU. Thank you for your encouragement, your confidence, your support, and your belief that I could do this – even when I doubted myself.

I know that God saw me as an author long before I did. I thank Him for helping me to stay rooted in scripture without knowing how He planned to use it in my story. I thank Him for the people He has coordinated to be a part of this project, and honestly, I thank Him for the people who have been part of my entire journey, even beyond that of a writer.

No one has supported me more than my husband, Richard. Words can never, ever express how much I love you, respect you, and acknowledge your role in helping me to become the woman that I was created to be. I thank you for being my teammate and best friend as we walk through life's adversities. I thank you for all of the nights you patiently allowed me to read each chapter, and your guidance in helping me to shape and narrate each challenge that we have faced regarding infertility. You are a blessing, and I am glad this journey has taught me not to neglect one blessing in pursuit of another. I love you so much and I'm honored to see where this experience leads us.

Much of this book would not have been possible without my mother. You provided the foundation to my understanding of how important it is to read the Bible and seek guidance in prayer. Thank you for demonstrating what it looks like to walk in faith and stand strong in conviction. And thank you for all of the discussions we shared while living on separate sides of the globe. Your pride and support for this project are wholeheartedly appreciated.

Thank you to my dear friends at Yoido English Ministry, especially Yoon and Rebecca Lee. You two already know how much of a fan I am of you and your dedication to the Gospel, but mostly I am incredibly grateful for your friendship and the pastoral care that you extended to Richard and myself during our time in Seoul. Thank you for providing the environment where we could continue to grow in spiritual maturity and embrace our responsibility in being "the Church". Richard and I have been blessed by you, and we look forward to reuniting with you in the future!

Thank you to all of the freelancers and test readers that helped to shape my idea from a simple document to a real book. I have such a big heart of gratitude for CJ as my awesome photographer and dear friend. Thank you for capturing "my good side" and for providing me with an abundance of photos to use for this project. Thanks to Ryan for listening to my ideas for the cover design, and your patience with my constant tweaks and modifications. Thank you, Rea, for ensuring the cohesiveness of the text and providing me with a final boost of confidence in tackling such a sensitive topic. Thank you to all of my beta readers for sharing your initial feedback, and being kind with constructive criticism. Thank you to Betsy and Sheri for your priceless words of praise and support.

There are a host of friends that I wish I could thank individually, but just know that I absolutely cherish your support. This project helped to highlight the depth of many of my relationships, and I do not take any of my family or friends for granted. I am especially grateful for the friends who have become mothers but did not shy away in supporting me with this topic. Thank you for your compassion with this subject, and for providing the space and gentle encouragement that I needed to process my thoughts and emotions. Thank you to the family and friends who have come to a place of sensitivity in realizing that everyone has a different story, a different journey, and a different ending. Thank you for respecting where Richard and I are on this journey.

And last, but most certainly not least, I want to acknowledge the women who have been afflicted by infertility but have not received the miracle. I know you have been forgotten and cast aside by society, but you do not go unnoticed by me. I thought about you as I wrote each chapter, and I prayed that I would say something that provided comfort or perspective for your experience. I am so sorry that there are so few resources that address the pain, struggle, and heartbreak that occurs when the miracle doesn't take place. It breaks my heart that there is such a strong stigma with infertility, especially as it applies to older women, women who do not have the opportunity to pursue advanced medical treatment, and families that have not been able to adopt. It hurts that this is part of the broken world that we live in, and that there is little that I can do to alleviate your pain. I hope that this book was just a small reminder that your circumstances do not make you "less than" anyone else. I hope it encourages you to lift your head higher and recognize that you are indeed seen and loved. I pray you find the strength to walk in confidence knowing that YOU...ARE... BLESSED.

Notes

RESOLVE: The National Infertility Association, "Fast Facts," resolve.org, February 2020, https://resolve.org/infertility-101/what-is-infertility/fast-facts.

Tyndale House Publishers. Study notes on Numbers. In *The Life Application Study Bible: New International Version*, 192-249. Carol Stream, IL: 2007

About the Author

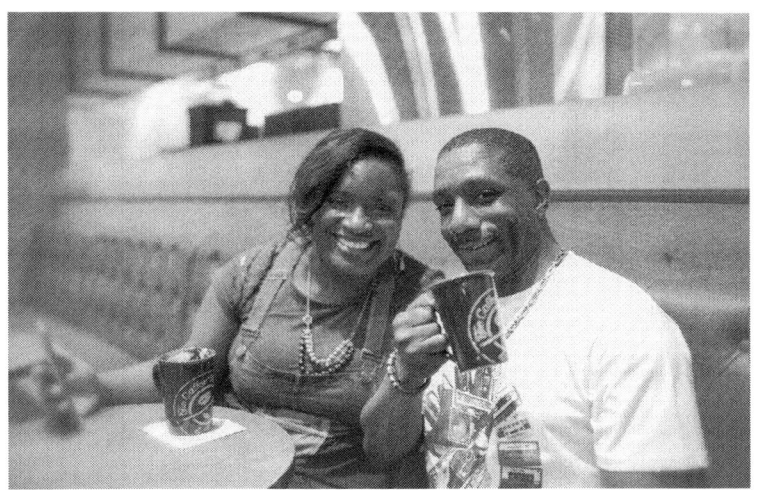

E rica Favors Mitchell is a native of Virginia and considers herself a learning aficionado. As a Certified Catalyst Facilitator for women's groups, she is passionate about pursuing personal growth and healing through reflection and acknowledging our need to grieve through loss. Erica personally enjoys quiet moments of contemplation and observation. As a Christian, she continually remains in awe of the depth of God's love and the profound measures that He will take to demonstrate His desire for a personal relationship with each of us. It is this inspiration that motivates her to appreciate the different cultural and ethnic diversities of the world. She enjoys making deep connections and developing meaningful relationships with persons of all backgrounds.

Her recent experiences have birthed an enthusiasm for international travel, and she has visited remote destinations in Southeast Asia—always selecting the window seat! International travel has matured her perspective on life, helping her to realize that difficult journeys often lead to unimaginable destinations.

Erica holds a B.A. in Sociology and is a graduate business student. She is relocating back to the United States after residing in South Korea with her husband, Richard, in devoted support of his career with the United States Navy.

You can connect with her on Facebook or Instagram (@nolessblessed) or at her website www.nolessbessed.com.

Made in the USA
Columbia, SC
07 February 2022

55670590R00080